THE TRUTH ABOUT
THE INTERNET AND
ONLINE PREDATORS

THE TRUTH ABOUT
THE INTERNET AND
ONLINE PREDATORS

Robert N. Golden, M.D.
University of Wisconsin-Madison
General Editor

Fred L. Peterson, Ph.D.
University of Texas-Austin
General Editor

Heath Dingwell, Ph.D.
Principal Author

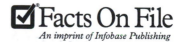

Facts On File
An imprint of Infobase Publishing

The Truth About the Internet and Online Predators

Facts On File, Inc.
An imprint of Infobase Publishing
132 West 31st Street
New York NY 10001

Library of Congress Cataloging-in-Publication Data

Dingwell, Heath.
   The truth about Internet and online predators / Robert N. Golden, general editor, Fred L. Peterson, general editor ; Heath Dingwell, principal author.
      p. cm.
   Includes bibliographical references and index.
   ISBN-13: 978-0-8160-7648-2 (hardcover : alk. paper)
   ISBN-10: 0-8160-7648-0 (hardcover : alk. paper) 1. Internet and teenagers. 2. Computer crimes. 3. Online sexual predators. 4. Internet. 5. Internet–Safety measures. I. Golden, Robert N. II. Peterson, Fred L. III. Title.
   HQ799.2.I5D56 2011
   004.67'80835–dc22
                                                    2010029296

Facts On File books are available at special discounts when purchased in bulk quantities for businesses, associations, institutions, or sales promotions. Please call our Special Sales Department in New York at (212) 967-8800 or (800) 322-8755.

You can find Facts On File on the World Wide Web at http://www.factsonfile.com

Excerpts included herewith have been reprinted by permission of the copyright holders; the author has made every effort to contact copyright holders. The publishers will be glad to rectify, in future editions, any errors or omissions brought to their notice.

Text design by David Strelecky
Composition by Kerry Casey
Cover printed by Yurchak Printing, Inc., Landisville, Pa.
Book printed and bound by Yurchak Printing, Inc., Landisville, Pa.
Date printed: April 2011
Printed in the United States of America

10 9 8 7 6 5 4 3 2 1

This book is printed on acid-free paper.

CONTENTS

LIST OF ILLUSTRATIONS

PREFACE

The Truth About series—updated and expanded to include 20 volumes—seeks to identify the most pressing health issues and social challenges confronting our nation's youth. Adolescence is the period between the onset of puberty and the attainment of adult roles and responsibilities. Adolescence is also a time of storm, stress, and risk-taking for many young people. During adolescence, a person's health is influenced by biological, psychological, and social factors, all of which interact with one's environment—family, peers, school, and community. It is a time when teenagers experience profound changes.

With the latest available statistics and new insights that have emerged from ongoing research, the Truth About series seeks to help young people build a foundation of information as they face some of the challenges that will affect their health and well-being. These challenges include high-risk behaviors, such as alcohol, tobacco, and other drug use; sexual behaviors that can lead to adolescent pregnancy and sexually transmitted diseases (STDs), such as HIV/AIDS; mental health concerns, such as depression and suicide; learning disorders and disabilities, which are often associated with school failures and school drop-outs; serious family problems, including domestic violence and abuse; and lifestyle factors, which increase adolescents' risk for noncommunicable diseases, such as diabetes and cardiovascular disease, among others.

Broader underlying factors also influence adolescent health. These include socioeconomic circumstances, such as poverty, available health care, and the political and social situations in which young people live. Although these factors can negatively affect adolescent health and well-being, as well as school performance, many of these negative health outcomes are preventable with the proper knowledge and information.

With prevention in mind, the writers and editors of each topical volume in the Truth About series have tried to provide cutting-edge information that is supported by research and scientific evidence. Vital facts are presented that inform youth about the challenges experienced during adolescence, while special features seek to dispel common myths and misconceptions. Some of the main topics explored include abuse, alcohol, death and dying, divorce, drugs, eating disorders, family life, fear and depression, rape, sexual behavior and unplanned pregnancy, smoking, and violence. All volumes discuss risk-taking behaviors and their consequences, healthy choices, prevention, available treatments, and where to get help.

In this new edition of the series, we also have added eight new titles in areas of increasing significance to today's youth. ADHD, or attention-deficit/hyperactivity disorder, and learning disorders are diagnosed with increasing frequency, and many students have observed or know of classmates receiving treatment for these conditions, even if they have not themselves received this diagnosis. Gambling is gaining currency in our culture, as casinos open and expand in many parts of the country, and the Internet offers easy access for this addictive behavior. Another consequence of our increasingly "online" society, unfortunately, is the presence of online predators. Environmental hazards represent yet another danger, and it is important to provide unbiased information about this topic to our youth. Suicide, which for many years has been a "silent epidemic," is now gaining recognition as a major public health problem throughout the life span, including the teenage and young adult years. We now also offer an overview of illness and disease in a volume that includes the major conditions of particular interest and concern to youth. In addition to illness, however, it is essential to emphasize health and its promotion, and this is especially apparent in the volumes on physical fitness and stress management.

It is our intent that each book serve as an accessible, authoritative resource that young people can turn for accurate and meaningful answers to their specific questions. The series can help them research particular problems and provide an up-to-date evidence base. It is also designed with parents, teachers, and counselors in mind so that they have a reliable resource that they can share with youth who seek their guidance.

Finally, we have tried to provide unbiased facts rather than subjective opinions. Our goal is to help elevate the health of the public with an emphasis on its most precious component—our youth. As young people face the challenges of an increasingly complex world, we as educators want them to be armed with the most powerful weapon available—knowledge.

Robert N. Golden, M.D.
Fred L. Peterson, Ph.D.
General Editors

HOW TO
USE THIS BOOK

NOTE TO STUDENTS

Knowledge is power. By possessing knowledge you have the ability to make decisions, ask follow-up questions, or know where to go to obtain more information. In the world of health that *is* power! That is the purpose of this book—to provide you with the power you need to obtain unbiased, accurate information and *The Truth About the Internet and Online Predators*.

Topics in each volume of The Truth About series are arranged in alphabetical order, from A to Z. Each of these entries defines its topic and explains in detail the particular issue. At the end of most entries are cross-references to related topics. A list of all topics by letter can be found in the table of contents or at the back of the book in the index.

How have these books been compiled? First, the publisher worked with me to identify some of the country's leading authorities on key issues in health education. These individuals were asked to identify some of the major concerns that young people have about such topics. The writers read the literature, spoke with health experts, and incorporated their own life and professional experiences to pull together the most up-to-date information on health issues, particularly those of interest to adolescents and of concern in Healthy People 2010.

Throughout the alphabetical entries, the reader will find sidebars that separate Fact from Fiction. There are Question-and-Answer boxes that attempt to address the most common questions that youths ask about sensitive topics. In addition, readers will find a special feature called "Teens Speak"—case studies of teens with personal stories related to the topic in hand.

This may be one of the most important books you will ever read. Please share it with your friends, families, teachers, and classmates. Remember, you possess the power to control your future. One way to affect your course is through the acquisition of knowledge. Good luck and keep healthy.

NOTE TO LIBRARIANS

This book, along with the rest of The Truth About series, serves as a wonderful resource for young researchers. It contains a variety of facts, case studies, and further readings that the reader can use to help answer questions, formulate new questions, or determine where to go to find more information. Even though the topics may be considered delicate by some, do not be afraid to ask patrons if they have questions. Feel free to direct them to the appropriate sources, but do not press them if you encounter reluctance. The best we can do as educators is to let young people know that we are there when they need us.

ONLINE BEHAVIOR: THE GOOD AND THE BAD

Over the past 20 years, the Internet has radically altered modern life. Chances are the Internet has played a role in your life for as long as you can remember. Generally, that is not a bad thing. People can buy almost anything online, and they can do so from the comfort of their homes. Web sites like Amazon.com are online "department stores" that provide customers with almost anything they want. EBay makes it easy to buy used items, usually directly from other customers. Priceline allows people to "name their own price" in an attempt to get the best plane, rental car, and hotel deals. The list goes on. As Jeff Jarvis, author of *What Would Google Do?,* said in a recent interview, "The Internet isn't a medium. . . . It's a place."

However, with the good comes the bad. The Internet is also used by some people to commit **identity theft,** find potential victims for ripoff scams, search for **child pornography,** try to meet children and teenagers for sex, and many more unsavory illegal behaviors. For every legitimate use of the Internet, there is no doubt an illegitimate one. To help readers avoid and recognize risky behaviors, this book will help explain the truth and many of the dangers associated with using the Internet.

RESEARCH ON INTERNET BEHAVIORS

Some Internet-related topics have been studied by many different researchers, making it relatively easy to gather information about them. Other topics, readers will notice, have received far less attention, making studying them challenging. The entry on physical threats over the Internet, for example, although a real danger, has received little to no attention by researchers. However, research on social networking Web sites and behavior has generated a great deal of documentation and data, making that topic easy to study. Until researchers have more time and funding, it may not be feasible to conduct research on relatively new topics.

Whenever possible, the latest research has been provided here. In some instances, however, older research is presented until such time as new studies become available.

THE SOCIAL IMPACT OF THE INTERNET ON DAILY LIFE

The Internet has done more than make many aspects of life easier. It also has changed the way people can interact with others. The exponential growth of social networking Web sites has made it easier to develop and maintain friendships, both local and long distance. Peoples' lives literally can be on display 24 hours a day, seven days a week. In addition to actually interacting with people in real time, it is possible to post updates on social networking Web sites. People can post updates all day and night, informing anyone from close friends to the whole world about their lives.

Cell phones also can be used to connect with Web sites, allowing the immediate posting of comments and pictures. Whether posting Twitter comments, pictures from a camera phone, or submitting updates to a social networking Web site, teenagers can keep "the world" up-to-date on all of their experiences.

Web sites have even started to pop up that focus on where people are located, as opposed to what they are doing. With the ability to track people becoming easier, there is one unintended yet very significant consequence. Thieves also can use this information to see if a person is at home. If a person indicates he or she is shopping, at the movies, or somewhere else, it means that person is not at home. That is one potential obstacle that thieves need not overcome if they want to break into someone's home.

INTERNET PREDATORS

One common concern among parents is that their child or teenager is being victimized by an Internet predator. One definition of a predator is a person who "victimizes, plunders, or destroys, especially for one's own gain." The term *predator* encompasses a wide range of offenders. For example, a cyber-bully can be viewed as an online predator because he or she victimizes others through demeaning and **abusive** comments or behavior. Identity thieves also can be viewed as predators because their goal is to steal the identities of others for personal gain. People who design **computer viruses** can be viewed as predators as well. However, the term *Internet predator* brings to mind another type of predator. That is the sexual predator, a sex offender who uses the Internet to find victims.

Sexual predators
It is difficult to say how many sexual predators are using the Internet to search and prey on children. Most of the research on Internet predators has focused on child pornographers. For example, a 2009 study in *Sexual Abuse: A Journal of Research and Treatment* examined the differences between child pornographers and offenders who had sexual contact with minors. The offenders who made contact had not approached the children over the Internet. Another 2009 study in the *Journal of the American Psychiatric Nurses Association* examined whether viewing pornography makes sexual offenders more dangerous. Although the focus was on sexual offenders, these offenders did not target children and teenagers over the Internet. Additional studies examine child pornographers, sexual offenders, and child molesters. However, because these studies do not necessarily focus on learning more about sexual offenders who rely on the Internet to find victims, gathering data is difficult.

Relative safety
Research does indicate, however, that most children and teenagers are pretty safe from Internet predators. Very few will make dates to meet strangers on the Internet. Although children and teenagers are exposed to sexual content on the Internet, only a fraction of young people are actively propositioned to meet someone in person for sex. Further, even fewer young people agree to such a meeting. This is a very important point to keep in mind. Undercover operations, whether conducted by the police or an investigative television program, are *actively* looking to meet predators in order to arrest them. Therefore, if a predator wants to meet, the undercover officer will arrange it. Most children do not want to meet and are unwilling to engage in sexual conversations with strangers.

Statistics on arrests

Arrest statistics show a significant difference when looking at predators arrested by an undercover officer versus those arrested after making physical contact with an actual child. The most reliable data comes from a 2009 report by the Crimes Against Children Research Center. The report indicates that between 2000 and 2006, there was a 381 percent increase in arrests when undercover agents posed as children. During the same period, there was a 21 percent increase in arrests when offenders made contact with children. Although there are offenders who are willing to meet children and teenagers for sex, the opportunity must present itself. Those opportunities are fewer when "real" children and teenagers are involved, as compared to the offenders' meeting with undercover officers.

The television show *To Catch a Predator* highlighted some of the potential dangers presented by online predators. This show revealed sting operations against the predators. People would pretend to be children and teenagers and talk with others on the Internet. If adults wanted to meet for sex, they would set up a day and time to meet. This meeting would take place at the "child's" house, where a camera crew and police officers waited. When the offender showed, he would be confronted and subsequently arrested. Watching this TV show resulted in many parents worrying if their children would be targeted by similar predators.

COMMONSENSE SURFING

Because the technology is still evolving and the statistics are being developed, there is some disagreement on what constitutes safe online behavior. Is it okay for people to know one's real name, address, e-mail, telephone number, and other contact information? Or should all of that be kept secret to protect one's privacy and safety? Common sense tells people to be very private and not share personal information. Realistically, however, privacy is contrary to why people use social networking. One of the main reasons people use the Internet is to interact with others. The questions everyone needs to ask are: What information should I share? Whom should I share it with? When should I share it?

THE INTERNET

Work on the Internet is said to have been started in 1969, when a computer scientist and his assistants at the University of California, Los Angeles, created the Advanced Research Projects Agency Network

(ARPANET). This project connected four universities over a network. By today's standards, this was a simple project, first connecting computers at UCLA, then making connections between UCLA and Stanford, and growing from there. At the time, however, the individuals and universities involved were considered pioneers. E-mail was introduced in 1972.

From the 1970s through the mid-1990s, the Internet and online world grew relatively slowly. In 1994, the White House launched its Web site. In 1995 alone, the following Web sites were launched: Yahoo, Amazon, eBay, and MSN. By 1996, there were approximately 45 million people using the Internet, with 75 percent of them residing in North America. Google was officially launched in 1998.

By 1999, there were approximately 150 million people using the Internet, more than a 300 percent increase in three years. Some estimates indicate that there were more than 300 million people using the Internet at that time. At the end of 2009, it was estimated that more than 1.8 billion people used the Internet worldwide. An estimated 90 trillion e-mails were sent during 2009. Approximately 72 trillion of those e-mails were spam.

RISKY BUSINESS SELF-TEST

The following questions are designed to measure the potential risks associated with your online behavior. For each question, answer true or false. Each time you answer "true," give yourself one point and record your answers on a separate sheet of paper. The higher the score, the riskier your online behavior is.

Chat room risks

____Do you tell people your first name in chat rooms?

____Do you tell people your last name in chat rooms?

____Do you publicly share your e-mail address in chat rooms?

____Do you publicly share your phone number in chat rooms?

____Do you publicly share your home address in chat rooms?

____Do you have sexual conversations in chat rooms with strangers?

___Do you try and pick fights (flaming) in chat rooms?

___Do you post pictures of yourself or friends in chat rooms?

Social networking risks

___Do you turn off your privacy settings?

___Can strangers access your personal information?

___Do you post potentially embarrassing or sexual pictures on your page?

___Do you post comments about your drinking, drug use, smoking, or sex life?

Instant messaging

___Do you IM with strangers?

___Do you have sexual conversations using IM?

___Do you share embarrassing or sexually explicit photos while using IM?

___Do you share personal information with strangers?

___Do you harass or bully people using IM?

General behavior

___Do you have an antivirus program running on your computer? [Answering "no" is considered a risky behavior.]

___Do you use an anti-spyware program? [Answering "no" is considered a risky behavior.]

___Is Internet monitoring or filtering software installed on your computer? [Answering "no" is considered a risky behavior.]

___Do you respond to e-mails that ask you for personal or account information?

___Do you download programs without paying for them?

___Do you download music without paying for it?

___Do you download videos without paying for them?

___Do you go to pornographic Web sites?

___Do you download pornography?

A–TO–Z ENTRIES

■ BLOGGING

Online tool for sharing information. Blogs are short for Weblogs. Anyone can start a blog and write about anything. A blog can be used as a personal diary, an information-sharing forum, a marketing or public relations tool, and more.

Teenagers typically use blogs to write about their personal lives. This sometimes includes writing about their sexual behaviors, drinking and drug use, parents, problems at school, and romantic relationships. Blogs are not very popular among teenagers, with only 8 percent blogging. Teens who blog often provide too much personal information, such as name, age, location, and e-mail address. Bloggers should take steps to protect their identity, such as using pseudonyms and not providing e-mail addresses or telephone numbers.

BLOGGING HISTORY

An article that appeared in a 2006 issue of *New York* magazine chronicled the early history of blogs. According to the author, the first blog was created in 1994 by a college student. The blog, Links. net, is still up and running. At that time the terms *Weblog* or *blog* did not exist. It was not until 1997 that the term *Weblog* was used, and in 1999, that was shortened to *blog*.

Blogging continued to grow, and by the beginning of 2005, it was estimated that more than 25 million people in the United States read blogs. There are at least 130 million blogs in existence today. However, it is difficult to tell how many blogs are active, meaning updated on a regular basis.

BASICS OF BLOGGING

Blogging allows a person to share as little or as much information as he or she wants. Blogging can be highly personal, sharing thoughts, feelings, and life experiences, or it can be used for professional purposes. In fact, one way job seekers boost their chances of success is by publishing informational pieces on a blog that publicizes their knowledge. A blog can be used to write about anything.

Searching blogs

One company, Technorati, is one of the world's leading sources of blogging information. According to the company's Web site, it is the leading **search engine** for blogs. Technorati collects information from millions of blogs and provides real-time search results for blog postings. A blogger can post something new to the blog and within minutes that post can be indexed by Technorati. Technorati does for blog searches what Google and Yahoo! do for Internet searches.

Technorati has become a social media company. Since 2004, it has published a "State of the Blogosphere" report. This report provides statistical information on blogs, including trends over the years, the types of people who use blogs, and so forth.

Who is blogging?

According to Technorati, 72 percent of bloggers do it for fun. They are considered hobbyists. This group is not concerned with making money from blogging. The next group is the part-timers, 15 percent of all bloggers. Part-timers try to make some money blogging. The next group is the self-employed, which makes up another 9 percent of bloggers. This group blogs full time. Of this group, 22 percent indicate that the blog is their business: Money is generated through the blog, often in the form of advertisements. Lastly, there are the corporate bloggers, who make up 4 percent of bloggers. This group writes blog material for companies. In a sense, it is a marketing or public relations job. These bloggers' goals are to spread news about a company, which will then attract people who want to do business with the company.

TEENS AND BLOGGING

Impression management is a key issue associated with blogging. Generally, the term refers to how a person presents herself or himself and the opinions people form based on that presentation. In blogging, a person's writing style and the information shared go a long way in forming others' impressions. As the authors of a 2010 article in the *Journal of Adolescent Research* note, blogs allow people to control their public persona.

This can be beneficial or problematic for bloggers. First, when blogs are public, as most are, anyone can read them. This includes people with good or bad intentions. An online predator, someone who intends to victimize someone else by demeaning or abusing that person online, can search those blogs that resemble the writings of a child or adolescent. Further, writing about drinking, drugs, or sexual behaviors also may catch the attention of predators. In a way, a blog can be viewed as a résumé in that it will attract certain people with an interest in the blogger.

Blogs as résumés

In a legitimate way, a blog and social networking information act as a résumé. Colleges, universities, and employers are searching the Internet to learn more about people. Someone who posts questionable material is less likely to be accepted into a program or offered employment. A Google or Yahoo! news search will show numerous articles where people have lost out on opportunities because of their objectionable postings.

Blogs can be customized. The user can configure background colors, layout, fonts, pictures, videos, border decorations, and more. These features also speak to the user's personality.

Nature of adolescents' blogs

A 2010 study in the *Journal of Adolescent Research* provided results on the content of blogs. The study authors focused on bloggers between the ages of 15 and 19. The authors found that 12.9 percent of bloggers discussed their sexuality and sexual behaviors. Almost 23 percent of bloggers discussed their romantic relationships. There were also blog entries that discussed alcohol and drug use. Slightly more than 44 percent of bloggers had posted pictures of themselves on their site.

The authors also found that while female bloggers seemed to focus more on themselves, friends, family, and significant others, male bloggers focused on less personal issues, such as society, celebrities, and other topics. This type of personal information can be used by online predators and offenders to victimize female bloggers.

Taken together, a predator can develop a good sense of what interests a blogger. For example, a young female blogger who discusses her relationships, sexual activity, and alcohol or drug use is providing the public with a wealth of information. Predators can use this type of personal information to strike up conversations and "connect" with the blogger.

The authors of a 2010 study in *Child and Adolescent Social Work Journal* had different findings. The authors studied blog postings from adolescents between the ages of 13 and 18. The posts were from the blog service Xanga. In contrast to other findings, the authors of this study noted that very few people mentioned sexual behavior. Approximately 1 percent mentioned something about sexuality in their posts. Most of the adolescents in this study discussed other activities, such as playing video games, watching television, computer

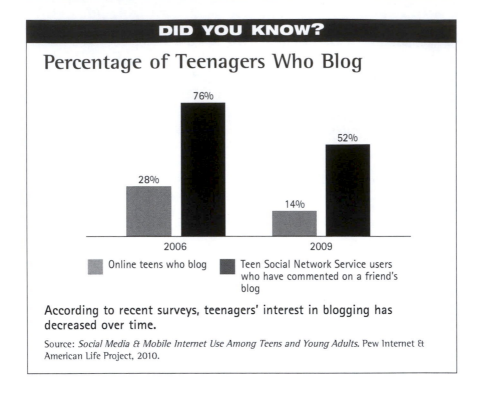

DID YOU KNOW?

Percentage of Teenagers Who Blog

According to recent surveys, teenagers' interest in blogging has decreased over time.

Source: *Social Media & Mobile Internet Use Among Teens and Young Adults.* Pew Internet & American Life Project, 2010.

use, and doing homework. However, the adolescents in this study also discussed their emotional states on the blogs. Slightly more than 56 percent indicated boredom, 30 percent mentioned feelings of depression, and 27.7 percent indicated feeling anger.

Discussing feelings is a great way to deal with stress. However, by posting this personal information on a blog, a blogger can become vulnerable. Readers can share their own experiences and feelings, thus establishing a bond between the blogger and readers. Predators or other online offenders can exploit this information and possibly victimize the blogger.

Too much personal information

The authors of a 2008 article in *Computers in Human Behavior* discuss the downfalls of providing too much personal information. They found that 55 percent of bloggers use their real name. As with other studies, the results here also indicated that bloggers tend to share personal information. Almost 82 percent of bloggers discussed themselves, while 68.2 percent discussed their relationships, and 72.7 percent discussed daily experiences.

A 2009 study in *CyberPsychology and Behavior* provides some evidence that bloggers are truthful with their entries. The authors of this study examined how often bloggers lied about personal information. The authors surveyed and interviewed bloggers between the ages of 13 and 17. The authors found that 34.5 percent of bloggers between the ages of 15 and 17 sometimes lied on their blogs. By comparison, 51.9 percent of younger bloggers (ages 13 and 14) sometimes lied on their blogs. When lying did occur, it was usually related to entries about relationships, skills, family situations, appearance, and sexual experience. The authors also noted that when younger bloggers lied about their sexual experience, they tended to exaggerate their experiences.

TEENS SPEAK

Blogging Is My Emotional Outlet

Blogging makes me feel better. It's hard to express myself because I'm shy around other people. That's not the case when I sit down and surf the Internet. I can do what I want without worrying what other people will think of me. It's the same thing when I'm blogging. No one knows my real identity, and I'm free to write whatever I want. I use Blogger, which is a free blog service from Google. I created a fake profile so people can't identify me. Anytime I write about things that happen in school I change everyone's name. The nice thing is I can write about my feelings and get feedback from other people. For me, I enjoy hearing about how other people go through the same things and what they do to deal with the problems. It's like going to a group therapy session, only it's free and anonymous.

There's only been a few times I've e-mailed or chatted with a person online after talking through a blog. I'm not a big fan of that since I'd rather people not know my real identity. That's easy to deal with. I can create a lot of different profiles for blogging, e-mail, and chatting. As long as

I'm careful, no one will really know who I am. Those conversations are nice, and no one has tried to hit on me yet. But for me, the most fun is through my blog. I don't know what I'd do without one anymore.

BLOGGING SAFETY TIPS

For teenagers who blog, it is important to remember some safety tips. According to the Electronic Frontier Foundation, a blogger should not give out any information that can help others identify the writer. Use a **pseudonym**. Do not mention the town you live in, where you go to school, or similar information. If someone does blog and wants to write about people or events, alter the information so it is more difficult for people to know the identity of the blogger.

Another safety option is to limit who can read the blog. Several blogging services allow users to protect the blog from the public. Only people who have been granted access can read the blog. This is similar to blogging on a social networking site, such as Facebook. Settings can be adjusted so only people in the person's social network can read material.

The corporation Microsoft advises bloggers not to post provocative pictures of themselves on a blog. If a user wants to remain truly anonymous then no identifying pictures should be posted. This includes avoiding pictures of the town in which you live, your friends, house, or school. There are documented cases where law enforcement officials have been able to track down predators across state lines just from looking at pictures, such as the inside of a hotel room.

Another tip from Microsoft is to consider anything you put on a blog to be permanent. Readers can save and print out copies of what a blogger writes. In the event that a blogger is identified, material may be used to embarrass or hurt the writer. Try to think not only of the present but also of the future.

See also: Chat Rooms and Instant Messaging; Internet Safety; Privacy Issues; Screen Names; Social Networking Web Sites

FURTHER READING
Bell, Ann. *Exploring Web 2.0: Second Generation Interactive Tools— Blogs, Podcasts, Wikis, Networking, Virtual Worlds, and More.* Scotts Valley, Calif.: CreateSpace, 2009.

Hussey, Tris. *Create Your Own Blog: 6 Easy Projects to Start Blogging Like a Pro.* Indianapolis, Ind.: Sams, 2010.

Selfridge, Benjamin, Peter Selfridge, and Jennifer Osborn. *A Teen's Guide to Creating Web Pages and Blogs.* Austin, Tex.: Prufrock Press, 2008.

■ BULLIES AND CYBER-BULLYING

Abusive online behavior. Bullies can use the Internet to act aggressively toward others. E-mail, social networking, and instant messaging allow bullies to pick on others any time of day or night. Studies show that between 11 and 57 percent of teenagers and young adults are victims of cyber-bullying.

Cyber-bullies also are likely to be victims. Most victims do not tell either parents or adults about being bullied. One of the most common reasons for this silence is fear that Internet privileges will be restricted.

FORMS OF CYBER-BULLYING

Cyber-bullying does not take place only through the Internet. Blogs, e-mail, instant messaging, and social networks all provide ways for abusive individuals to bully people. Even **text messaging** by cell phone can be a form of cyber-bullying.

According to the authors of a 2008 study in the *Journal of School Health,* insults appear to be the most common form of cyber-bullying. Insults are followed by threats, stealing passwords, sharing private information, and sending or posting embarrassing pictures.

The authors of a 2009 article in *New Media & Society* present characteristics of both traditional and online bullying. According to the writers, traditional bullying involves physical or verbal actions, social exclusion, and property damage. The authors also reference indirect bullying, which focuses on spreading rumors.

Like traditional bullying, cyber-bullying also includes aspects of direct and indirect bullying. For example, property can be damaged by sending viruses. Verbal threats and insults can occur through both telephones and instant messaging programs that have a voice option. Bullies also can attempt to exclude people from talking with other people in social networks or chat groups. The Internet also allows for a variety of indirect bullying tactics, such as sharing personal e-mails, spreading rumors, and creating Web pages or voting polls designed to humiliate someone.

The authors of a 2009 article in *New Media & Society* indicate that some cyber-bullying may be accidental. The point is well taken, because purely electronic forms of communication can be misinterpreted. Someone may make a joke or sarcastic comment that is then interpreted as a threat or intimidating remark. The best way to determine if comments are threatening in nature is to ask the sender.

TEENS SPEAK

I Thought I Could Relax at Home.

It was bad enough that I would get picked on at school. I was always being called fat, ugly, and a slut. It didn't matter how hard I tried to fit in or ignore the comments. They just kept coming. At least I could look forward to enjoying myself when I got home. Then the bullies took that away as well. I would get e-mails making fun of me. Someone designed a Web site that made fun of me. Apparently people made fun of me on MySpace or Facebook—I can't remember which one. I changed my e-mail address, and no one from school has it. I don't pay attention to any of the social networking sites. It would just be nice if people would leave me alone. It's not like I did anything to them. I wish they would find better things to do with their time.

PREVALENCE OF CYBER-BULLYING

Researchers disagree about the extent of cyber-bullying. The authors of a 2009 article in the *Journal of Educational Administration* conducted a survey of first- and second-year college students in order to learn more about cyber-bullying. They found that:

- 56.1 percent of the students surveyed had experienced cyber-bullying
- 72.1 percent of females had been victimized, while only 27.9 percent of males reported being victimized

Authors of a 2009 article in the journal *School Psychology International* found that only 9 percent of middle schools students, ages 11 through 15, had received a threatening message that made them afraid. However, 35 percent of the students indicated that they had occasionally received a threatening message. Between 3 percent and 7 percent of students indicated they often receive such messages, which is more consistent with notions about bullying.

A 2008 article found in the *Journal of School Health* indicates that cyber-bullying may be common among youth. The authors collected information on students between the ages of 12 and 17. They found that 72 percent of students experienced at least one incident of cyber-bullying in the past year. However, only 19 percent of students were victims of repeated cyber-bullying, which was defined as having experienced at least seven incidents during the prior year.

In a 2009 article found in *New Media & Society,* the authors surveyed almost 1,100 students between the ages of 10 and 18 years old. Only 11.1 percent of the students said they had been victims of cyber-bullying; 18 percent admitted to engaging in cyber-bullying. The most common forms of bullying were making insults or threats, pretending to be the victim (deception), and spreading gossip.

An article in a 2008 issue of the *Scandinavian Journal of Psychology* examined cyber-bullying among students ages 12 through 20. Similar to the study in *New Media & Society* referenced above, only 11.7 percent of students indicated they had been victims of cyber-bullying. Students between the ages of 12 and 15 were more likely to be victims, with 17.6 percent of this group being cyberbullied. By comparison, only 3.3 percent of those between the ages of 15 and 20 reported having been victims of cyber-bullying.

Q & A

Question: Is suicide related to being cyberbullied?

Answer: According to a 2010 fact sheet published by the Cyberbullying Research Center, cyber-bullying can increase the risk of someone thinking about or attempting suicide. The authors of the fact sheet indicate that cyber-bullying victims were 1.9 times more likely to attempt suicide than non-victims. Victims of traditional bullying were 1.7 times more likely to attempt suicide than non-victims.

CYBER-BULLIES

It can be difficult to learn the characteristics of cyber-bullies. Unlike traditional bullying where a victim can identify the bully, cyber-bullies can make up a set of characteristics. For example, the authors of the previously cited 2008 article in *Scandinavian Journal of Psychology* noted that 36.2 percent of the victims did not know the gender of an online bully.

Authors of a 2009 article in *School Psychology International* found that approximately 25 percent of students in their survey engaged in cyber-bullying. The most commonly stated reason for cyber-bullying was disliking the victim. The second most cited reason was that the victim upset them.

Findings in a 2007 article published in *Developmental Psychology* indicate that text messaging was the most common form of cyber-bullying. According to the authors, 32.1 percent of victims were harassed through text messages.

CHARACTERISTICS OF VICTIMS

Authors of a 2009 article in *Social Work Research* examined a sample of Web posts by children and youth that were written on a counseling Web site. The samples dealt with Internet relationships involving issues of abuse. When girls were targets of bullying, the bullies typically made fun of the girls' weight. Sexual orientation was another area of attack, for both boys and girls.

In a 2007 issue of *Developmental Psychology,* the authors of an article studied the relationship between traditional bullying and electronic bullying. Of the 41 students who were victims of electronic bullying, the authors found that 35 of them (85 percent) were also victims of traditional bullying.

The authors of a 2009 article in the *Journal of Educational Administration* found that 91 percent of cyber-bullying incidents were a result of relationship problems. The authors also found that females would receive messages attacking appearance or popularity. Conversely, the focus of messages toward males targeted sexual orientation.

Victims of cyber-bullying are also likely to be cyber-bullies themselves. Authors of a 2009 study in the *Journal of Media Psychology* found that those who engaged in both traditional and cyber-bullying were also victims of these types of bullying. The authors also discovered that victims often went to Internet sites that could be considered

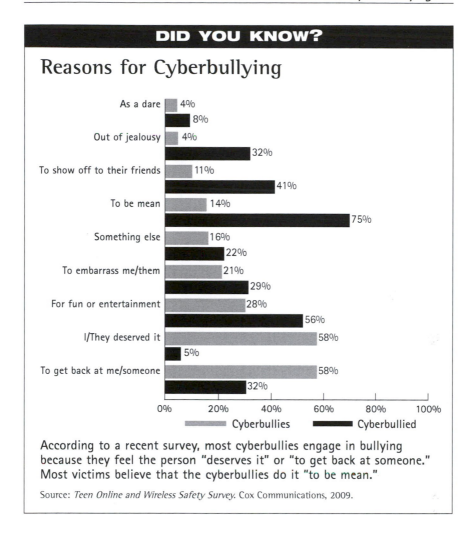

DID YOU KNOW?

Reasons for Cyberbullying

As a dare — 4% / 8%
Out of jealousy — 4% / 32%
To show off to their friends — 11% / 41%
To be mean — 14% / 75%
Something else — 16% / 22%
To embarrass me/them — 21% / 29%
For fun or entertainment — 28% / 56%
I/They deserved it — 58% / 5%
To get back at me/someone — 58% / 32%

Cyberbullies   Cyberbullied

According to a recent survey, most cyberbullies engage in bullying because they feel the person "deserves it" or "to get back at someone." Most victims believe that the cyberbullies do it "to be mean."

Source: *Teen Online and Wireless Safety Survey.* Cox Communications, 2009.

risky. These included extremist and pornographic chat rooms, which are conducive to verbal abuse. Instances of bullying may be a reflection of the norms associated with the chat room instead of being a personal attack against someone. In other words, such abusive behavior may be expected from people who enter these chat rooms.

HANDLING CYBER-BULLYING

The authors of a 2008 article in *Scandinavian Journal of Psychology* also found that 50 percent of victims did not tell anyone, including friends, about having been bullied. None of the students ever reported an incident to their teachers, while only 8.9 percent told a parent or guardian.

Fear of the consequences

As with traditional bullying, victims often will not report the problem to parents or teachers. Authors of a 2009 article in the *Journal of Educational Administration* found that only 35.9 percent of victims told their parents. Further, only 16.7 percent of victims informed school officials. Many victims were afraid how their parents would react, including the possibility of punishing them. Victims also lacked confidence that school officials would either take the problem seriously or handle it in a way that did not cause even more problems.

Authors of a 2009 article in *School Psychology International* asked students if they reported the incidents to anyone. The authors found that 74 percent would tell their friends, while 57 percent indicated they would tell a parent. However, only 42 percent would tell a school official. The most common reasons for not involving school officials were:

- fear of retaliation by the bully
- it's not the school's problem
- the school staff could not stop the bully

Approximately 24 percent of students also indicated fear of having their Internet access restricted by their parents.

This information contrasts with data reported on in a 2008 article in the *Journal of School Health.* In that article, the authors found that 90 percent of students would not tell adults about the incidents. The most common response was students felt they needed to learn to deal with the problem themselves. However, 31 percent also indicated they feared their Internet access would be restricted by telling their parents.

Similarities to traditional bullying

Both traditional bullying and cyber-bullying can have significant consequences for the victims. The authors of a 2009 article in the *Journal of Educational Administration* found that victims of cyber-bullying experienced several psychological effects. In particular, victims experienced fear, sadness, powerlessness, and anger. Further, it was found that these feelings were even stronger when a person did not know the identity of the bully.

Similar results were obtained by the authors of a 2009 article in *Social Work Research*. The authors found that victims of bullying experienced "feelings of depression, confusion, guilt, and shame as well as self-harm and withdrawal from peers and family."

See also: Chat Rooms and Instant Messaging; Internet Safety; Online Victimization, Examples of; Peers and Peer Pressure; Prejudice and Online Behavior; Prevention and Statistics

FURTHER READING

McQuade III, Samuel C., James P. Colt, and Nancy Meyer. *Cyber Bullying: Protecting Kids and Adults From Online Bullies.* Santa Barbara, Calif.: Praeger, 2009.

Shariff, Shaheen. *Confronting Cyber-Bullying: What Schools Need to Know to Control Misconduct and Avoid Legal Consequences.* New York: Cambridge University Press, 2009.

Trolley, Barbara C., and Constance Hanel. *Cyber Kids, Cyber Bullying, Cyber Balance.* Thousand Oaks, Calif.: Corwin, 2009.

■ CHAT ROOMS AND INSTANT MESSAGING

These are online opportunities for and methods of real-time communications. Chat rooms and instant messaging services allow people to have online conversations. These forms of communication are popular among children and teenagers and also lend themselves to cyber-bullying, online predators, and **software** attacks. In particular, instant messaging is a popular tool used for cyber-bullying, and predators use this method to make contact with potential victims.

CHAT ROOMS

Unlike blogging and social networking Web sites, chat rooms and instant messaging software allow people to interact with each other in "real time." There is no delay.

Research shows that chat rooms are popular among children and teenagers. Authors of a study in a 2008 issue of the *Journal of School Health* examined cyber-bullying behavior, which included bullying in chat rooms. The authors found that 59 percent of the children in the study used chat rooms. However, only 6 percent experienced bullying in chat rooms. According to reports, cyber-bullies are more likely to use text messaging and instant messaging to victimize others.

TEENS SPEAK

Chat Rooms Are Just for Fun

Personally, I don't know what the big deal is about chat rooms being dangerous. They are just for fun. You're going to run into all sorts of weirdos in these places. That's part of the reason it's fun—you get to mess around with these people. My friends and I will get together and go into these rooms just to mess around. You find these people who seem to devote their lives to online chatting. And then there are the sickos who want to talk about sex. Sometimes we'll pretend to be innocent and play along. Then we'll tell the guy that we're an old guy just messing around. That really gets people mad. But what's someone going to do? We don't use our real names and certainly don't tell the truth about who we are or where we live. Why would anyone want to do that? You can't trust people you meet in a chat room. That's why I just chat for fun. No harm, no foul.

Types of chat rooms

There are thousands of chat rooms on the Internet. These include free and paid, members only, rooms. Chat rooms offer more anonymity than other "conversations" as they tend to be text-based. There are usually no audio or video features. When there are dozens of people in a room it can be difficult to follow all conversations. There may only be a couple of people chatting or dozens of people vying for each others' attention. Add audio or video to that, and it would be impossible to make sense of everything going on.

Avatar

A growing feature of chat rooms is the use of an **avatar.** These are graphical representations of a user. Avatars can be real photos of a person, a symbol, or a computer-generated character. Online games such as World of Warcraft and Second Life use avatars to represent players. Unfortunately, avatars used in a chat room can help bullies or predators identify their targets, and avatars designed to represent something sexual will be especially appealing to sexual predators. Cyber-bullies also use this graphic information to make fun of other users. Demeaning the avatar or what it represents can be hurtful if a person truly believes the avatar represents his or her identity.

Chat rooms and sexual predators

There have been numerous cases in which chat rooms were used to lure kids and teenagers into sexual situations. In 2005, Yahoo! shut down its Teen Chat Room service. The company discovered that these chat rooms were being used to facilitate sex between children and adults. The company Security Software Systems indicates that predators do not try to seduce children in chat rooms. Instead, they use chat rooms as a hunting ground. When possible, the offender tries to make initial contact by instant message.

Looking for partners

Authors of a 2007 article in *CyberPsychology and Behavior* examined teen chat rooms to see how users looked for partners. The authors examined 12,000 comments in chat rooms that were both monitored and unmonitored. Almost 11 percent of all comments were requests for partners. These requests came from 53 percent of participants. The authors found virtually no difference in the number of partner requests between monitored versus unmonitored chat rooms (10.9 percent versus 10.7 percent).

Even fewer partner requests were of a sexual nature. Only 1.9 percent of requests in monitored rooms and 2.0 percent of requests in unmonitored rooms fell into this category. Even fewer requests still involved asking for a picture. Only 0.3 percent in monitored rooms and 0.8 percent in unmonitored rooms indicated requests for pictures.

INSTANT MESSAGING

There are several instant messaging programs available. These include Yahoo! Messenger, AOL Instant Messenger, Apple's iChat, ICQ, Windows Live Messenger, and Google Talk. There are also programs that allow the user to access several instant messaging services at once. Many users use more than one instant messenger. To make life easier, there are programs that allow users to log in to each of their instant messengers at the same time without having to start up each program.

One example is Trillian Astra. This program permits a user to chat on Windows Live, MySpace IM, Yahoo!, Google, ICQ, Jabber, IRC, and Skype. The software also allows a user to manage his or her e-mail, Facebook, and Twitter accounts. In a sense it is the ultimate convenience program for social networking. The software also lets users have audio and video chats.

Social networking Web sites such as Facebook also have instant messaging capabilities. Such features on social networks have proven to be popular. For example, in June 2009 Facebook announced that more than 1 billion instant messages were being sent each day.

Instant messaging software can take real-time interaction even further than chat rooms. Depending on the program used, people can use audio and video. Although a person cannot completely see the other person, new software allows users to interact as if they were physically next to each other.

Good and bad consequences

This has both positive and negative consequences. On the positive side, deception is extremely difficult when you can see and hear the other person. An older male claiming to be a teenager will not be able to pull that off when audio and video are used. However, audio and video add a more personal dimension to harassment and abuse.

Instant messaging offers bullies another way to harass victims. Findings in a 2007 article published in *Developmental Psychology* indicated that text messaging was the most common form of cyberbullying. Although not done through the Internet, text messaging is a form of instant messaging. According to the authors, 32.1 percent of victims were harassed through text messages.

Other dangers of IMs and texts

Another potential danger of instant messaging is receiving files containing **viruses, spyware,** or some other form of **malware.** In 2009, a Trojan Horse virus called Zeus infected approximately 3.6 million computers through instant messaging. The virus collected banking information and sent it to the offender. Even worse, although many of the infected computers had up-to-date antivirus protection, the Zeus still managed to obtain sensitive information.

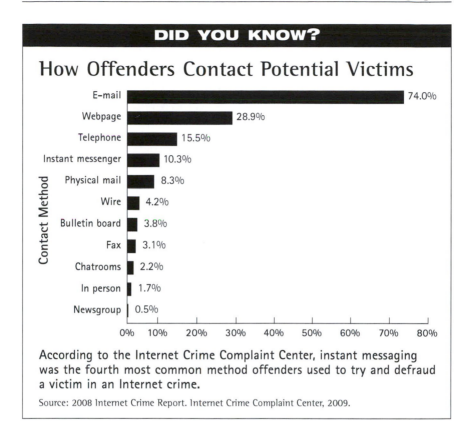

DID YOU KNOW?

How Offenders Contact Potential Victims

According to the Internet Crime Complaint Center, instant messaging was the fourth most common method offenders used to try and defraud a victim in an Internet crime.

Source: 2008 Internet Crime Report. Internet Crime Complaint Center, 2009.

A 2009 annual report produced by MessageLabs, a part of the antivirus program Symantec, indicates that instant messaging threats will continue to grow. According to the company, instant messaging will be threatened by **spam** that contains malicious links. Another issue mentioned by MessageLabs is friend-phishing. This occurs when a person's username and password for the instant messaging program are compromised. As a result, instant messages are sent to users on a contact list. The message directs the person to a Web site, where malicious code is used to obtain the victim's username and password for the IM program. This cycle continues to perpetuate itself.

In 2009, Google's instant messaging service, Google Talk, was the target of a phishing scheme. Users were receiving messages with instructions to check out a Web site. If a user tried to visit the Web site, he or she was informed their Google Talk username and password were needed to access the site. Entering this information then compromised the person's account.

See also: Internet Safety; Online Victimization, Examples of; Phishing and Pharming; Privacy Issues

FURTHER READING
Bridgewater, Rachel, and Meryl B. Cole. *Instant Messaging Reference: A Practical Guide.* Oxford, U.K.: Chandos Publishing, 2009.
Stern, Shayla Thiel. *Instant Identity: Adolescent Girls and the World of Instant Messaging.* New York: Peter Lang Publishing, 2007.

■ CYBER-BULLYING
See: Bullies and Cyber-bullying

■ CYBER-CRIMES AND LAW ENFORCEMENT
Regulations imposed by authorities in response to Internet crime. Cyber-crimes are a growing problem and can quickly overwhelm the resources of law enforcement agencies. Cyber-crime units exist within local, state, federal, and international law enforcement agencies. The Federal Bureau of Investigation (FBI) plays a critical role in investigating crimes committed through the Internet. Other organizations, such as Carnegie Mellon University's Computer Emergency Response Team, provide help to law enforcement and businesses to combat and control cyber-crimes.

CYBER-CRIME OVERVIEW
According to the U.S. Department of Justice, there are several types of cyber-crime. These include computer intrusion, password trafficking, counterfeiting of currency, child pornography or exploitation, Internet fraud and spam, Internet harassment, Internet bomb threats, and using or trafficking explosive or incendiary devices or firearms over the Internet. Other crimes include copyright piracy, trademark counterfeiting, and theft of trade secrets.

According to a 2010 report by the firm Deloitte, there are several worrisome trends, including

1. An increase in cyber-attacks and security breaches
2. Cyber-criminals using technological innovations faster than organizations can keep up
3. Cyber-defense techniques, such as virus protection and perimeter-intrusion detection, rapidly becoming outdated

Difficulty catching criminals

Catching cyber-criminals can be difficult. One problem is determining which law enforcement agency has jurisdiction over a case. Does the agency where the offender lives pursue a case? Or does the agency where the victim lives lead the investigation? If a cyber-crime occurs over state lines, then federal authorities need to get involved.

Other law enforcement problems

The authors of a 2009 article published in *Policing: An International Journal of Police Strategies & Management* highlight some other law enforcement issues. These include properly collecting evidence, deciding how to apply current laws to cyber-crimes, and detecting cyber-criminals.

FEDERAL BUREAU OF INVESTIGATION

The FBI maintains a cyber-unit for investigating cyber-crimes. According to the FBI's Web site, their cyber-unit has four missions. These are

1. To stop those behind the most serious computer intrusions and the spread of malicious code
2. To identify and thwart online sexual predators who use the Internet to meet and exploit children and to produce, possess, or share child pornography
3. To counteract operations that target U.S. intellectual property, endangering our national security and competitiveness
4. To dismantle national and transnational organized criminal enterprises engaging in Internet fraud

Operation Phish Phry

In October 2009, the FBI concluded a two-year investigation called Operation Phish Phry. The FBI worked with Egyptian authorities and

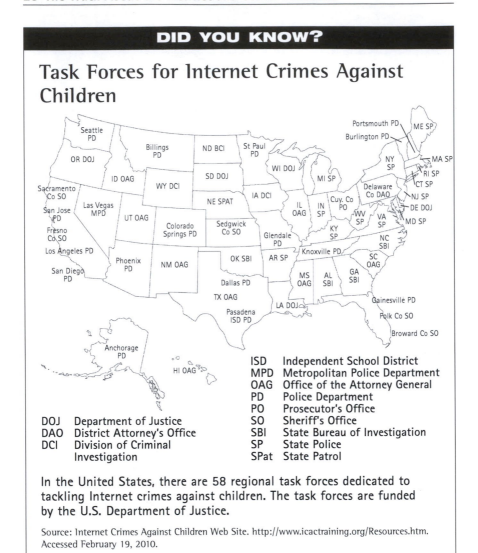

DID YOU KNOW?

Task Forces for Internet Crimes Against Children

ISD Independent School District
MPD Metropolitan Police Department
OAG Office of the Attorney General
PD Police Department
PO Prosecutor's Office
SO Sheriff's Office
SBI State Bureau of Investigation
SP State Police
SPat State Patrol

DOJ Department of Justice
DAO District Attorney's Office
DCI Division of Criminal Investigation

In the United States, there are 58 regional task forces dedicated to tackling Internet crimes against children. The task forces are funded by the U.S. Department of Justice.

Source: Internet Crimes Against Children Web Site. http://www.icactraining.org/Resources.htm. Accessed February 19, 2010.

arrested 100 suspects. Fifty-three of the suspected cyber-criminals were charged in the United States. The goal of the investigation was to disrupt a sophisticated attempt by the group to illegally use the financial accounts of potential victims.

Phishing is the attempt to gather sensitive information, such as usernames, passwords, credit card numbers, and other financial information. Potential victims receive an e-mail that claims to be from their bank or credit card company. That e-mail directs them to a Web site, which is designed to look like their banking or credit card Web site, where the victim is asked to enter account information for verification purposes. That information can then be used for illegal personal gain, such as emptying another person's bank accounts.

The phishing attacks originated in Egypt, which is why the FBI enlisted the help of Egyptian authorities. All defendants were accused to commit wire fraud and bank fraud. Individual defendants were charged with a variety of offenses, including aggravated identity theft, conspiracy to commit computer fraud, and both domestic and international money laundering. As of March 2010, the case was still proceeding through the courts.

STATE CYBER-CRIME UNITS

There are cyber-crime units in all 50 states. Some of these units may be operated by a state organization, such as the state police. Other units may be multi-jurisdictional, involving local, state, and even federal officials. Some states even have several units, which may be found at the local and state levels.

New York State maintains several cyber-crime units. One such unit is the New York State Office of Cyber Security and Critical Infrastructure Coordination (CSCIC). The unit works with all levels of government, as well as with the private and public sectors, to coordinate prevention and response activities to cyber-crimes.

The CSCIC conducts red team attacks, the goal of which is to gain control of someone else's system. In other words, the goal is to hack into a computer network. Performing such an attack allows the unit to see what vulnerabilities exist. Identify the vulnerabilities and the proper measures can be taken to fix them. The CSCIC is also responsible for intrusion detection and response. They monitor state systems to make sure no hacking attempts or suspicious activity is occurring. When cyber-attacks occur, the CSCIC can coordinate the response.

Another example of a state agency is the Maine State Police Computer Crimes Unit. This unit assists law enforcement with criminal investigations that involved the use of computers. They have assisted in homicides, drug trafficking, harassment, and domestic violence cases. However, the unit's priority is to focus on cases of Internet child exploitation. Thanks to federal funding, the unit has been able to hire additional full-time investigators to help track down child pornographers.

The Maine Computer Crimes Unit made headlines around the country in 2008 when it helped track down a child pornographer. Authorities from Australia had contacted the FBI about a group of child pornography traders. The investigation worked its way to Maine. After an arrest was made in Maine, one of the investigators from the Maine unit started examining pictures to gather clues about the offender. The investigator analyzed clues from 1,800 videos and pictures to track the offender to Georgia, where he was arrested and subsequently confessed to the crimes. Examples like this demonstrate the potential complexity of cyber-crimes. They are not confined to one geographical area, which means that multiple law enforcement agencies often have to work together.

INTERPOL

INTERPOL, The International Criminal Police Organization, is the world's largest police organization. INTERPOL has 188 member countries. INTERPOL helps law enforcement agencies around the world share information. Member countries can access INTERPOL's communications system that allows law enforcement agencies to post and retrieve data. Available data include fingerprints, information on suspected terrorists, DNA profiles, lost or stolen documents, wanted criminals lists, and much more. Each nation maintains its own database of information. Through INTERPOL, member nations can access each other's databases.

INTERPOL and crisis response

INTERPOL also provides crisis response services to member countries. If a disaster or major crime is committed, INTERPOL can assemble and deploy a crisis response team within hours. This team will then provide support and help coordinate activities as needed.

INTERPOL and cyber-crimes

INTERPOL works with organizations and private companies around the world to help prevent and investigate cyber-crimes. INTERPOL's cyber-crime efforts include dealing with copyright piracy, product counterfeiting (for example, fake medications), money counterfeiting, money laundering, and financial fraud, such as phishing scams.

Ironically, even INTERPOL has been targeted in phishing schemes. In 2006, a false INTERPOL Web site was created, and the offenders sent e-mails to potential victims. The e-mails directed people to go to the Web site where they then would be asked to provide sensitive information.

Fact Or Fiction?

Downloading music is not a crime.

The Facts: It is legal to **download** some music. The music must be in the **public domain,** meaning it is not protected by copyright laws. Some singers and bands freely distribute their music for listening. If a singer or band does not freely distribute their work, then people need to pay to download the music.

Downloading music without paying for it is a crime. It is referred to as music piracy. The Recording Industry Association of America estimates that more than $12 billion is lost per year because of music piracy. People who were accused of illegally **uploading** and downloading music were being arrested and taken to court. However, the RIAA has now switched tactics and is working with Internet service providers to stop people from illegally sharing music.

COMPUTER EMERGENCY RESPONSE TEAM (CERT)

Cyber-crime is such a widespread problem that law enforcement agencies cannot handle all of it. Other organizations exist to assist law enforcement agencies and both public and private companies in trying to control cyber-crimes. One such organization is the Computer Emergency Response Team, which is operated out of Carnegie Mellon University in Pittsburgh, Pennsylvania. According to the CERT Web site, the CERT mission is to

1. Provide a reliable, trusted, 24-hour, single point of contact for emergencies
2. Facilitate communication among experts working to solve security problems
3. Serve as a central point for identifying and correcting vulnerabilities in computer systems
4. Maintain close ties with research activities and conduct research to improve the security of existing systems
5. Initiate proactive measures to increase awareness and understanding of information security and computer

security issues throughout the community of network users and service providers

In 1988, the Morris Worm Incident occurred. A worm is a program that can run and spread by itself. Unlike a virus, it does not need to attach itself to files that are shared among users. The worm spread like wildfire and caused approximately $98 million in damages. Approximately 6,000 systems were infected. In 1988, this accounted for 10 percent of all Internet-capable computers.

Because of the devastating consequences of this worm, several initiatives were taken to help prevent and stop future attacks. Many people consider CERT to be the premier organization to deal with cyber-crimes.

One of CERT's objectives is to analyze the state of Internet security and then distribute the findings online. They analyze areas of vulnerability for organizations and help design remedies for those weaknesses. Similarly, CERT also analyzes software vulnerabilities. By identifying vulnerabilities, software patches can be designed to help prevent security breaches. CERT also helps companies develop computer security incident response teams. These teams respond to security threats and breaches. They are among the types of responders who have evolved to aid law enforcement in this growing area of criminal activity.

See also: Hate Crimes and Online Predators; Internet Safety; Laws Against Online Predators; Phishing and Pharming; Privacy Issues

FURTHER READING

Dhanjani, Nitesh, Billy Rios, and Brett Hardin. *Hacking: The Next Generation.* Sebastopol, Calif.: O'Reilly, 2009.

Kramer, Franklin D., Stuart H. Starr, and Larry Wentz. *Cyberpower and National Security.* Dulles, Va.: Potomac Books, 2009.

Menn, Joseph. *Fatal System Error: The Hunt for the New Crime Lords Who Are Bringing Down the Internet.* Jackson, Tenn.: PublicAffairs, 2010.

■ CYBER-TERRORISM

See: Cyber-crimes and Law Enforcement

■ FACEBOOK
See: Prevalence and Statistics; Social Networking Web Sites

■ FRIENDSTER
See: Prevalence and Statistics; Social Networking Web Sites

■ GENDER AND ONLINE PREDATORS
Differences in male and female behavior in online abusive situations. Research has shown some gender differences in online predatory behavior. Although approximately 4 percent of all online sexual offenders are female, there have been no documented cases of females being arrested as online predators. Research has focused exclusively on men. However, both girls and boys engage in cyber-bullying. Whereas boys are more likely to be the bullies, girls are more likely to be the victims. Gender differences also exist when it comes to online privacy issues. Males are less concerned than females about privacy and, as a result, they share more personal information online.

GENDER AND SEXUAL PREDATORS
Online sexual predators are almost always male. There has not been any research examining online female predators. The reason is simple: Females are not arrested for online predatory behavior. Further, there is very little research on female sexual offenders in general. The authors of a 2009 article in the *Journal of Family Violence* reported that female sexual offenders are "little studied and poorly understood." They go on to indicate that between 1989 and 2004, a span of 15 years, only 13 studies on female sexual offenders were published, which had a sample size of at least 10 offenders. As a result, the ability to generalize such findings to female sexual offenders is very difficult.

The Canadian Children's Rights Council estimates that 25 percent of sexual predators are women. However, that figure is likely to be overestimated. The authors of an article in a 2010 issue of the *Archives of Sexual Behavior* say that only 4 to 5 percent of *all* sexual offenses are committed by women.

Female sexual offenders often target children and teenagers. Authors of a 2009 article in the *Journal of Family Violence* reviewed studies on female sexual offenders. According to the authors, one study found that 53 percent of victims were between the ages of 12 and 17. Another study found 67.7 percent of victims were between 12 and 17. Yet another study indicated that 50 percent of victims were between 11 and 16, while still another study found that 24 percent were between ages four and 10.

Fact Or Fiction?

Boys and girls are at equal risk of being victimized by an online sexual predator.

The Facts: Girls are more likely than boys to be targets of online sexual predators. The authors of a 2008 study in *American Psychologist* looked at these gender differences. Their review indicated that girls, especially those who are sexually active, are more at risk than boys to be victims of online sexual predators. Approximately 75 percent of victims of Internet-initiated sex crimes are girls. The authors also found that boys who are victims are more likely to be gay or have questions about their sexuality.

Why so little research on women?
Some research provides a clue as to why there is no data for online female predators. In a 2009 article found in the *Journal of Family Violence,* the authors indicated that female offenders typically know their victims. There is no need to search the Internet for victims. Reviewing numerous studies, the authors found that between 45.5 and 68 percent of child victims were biologically related female offenders. Typically the victim was the offender's child. The authors of a 2009 article in *Criminal Justice and Behavior* also stated that female offenders are more likely than male offenders to victimize relatives.

A 2009 report by the Administration for Children and Families, part of the U.S. Department of Health and Human Services, found that 38.7 percent of child abuse victims were abused by the mother. Almost 18 percent of victims were abused by the father.

Some conclusions
The research is not definitive regarding gender differences for online sexual offenders, because the online behaviors of female sexual

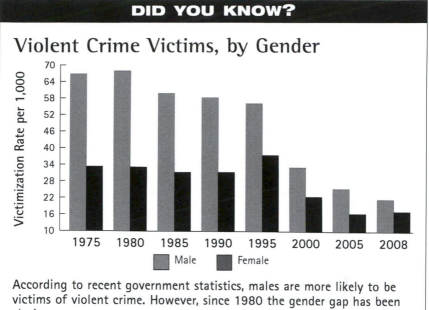

DID YOU KNOW?

Violent Crime Victims, by Gender

According to recent government statistics, males are more likely to be victims of violent crime. However, since 1980 the gender gap has been closing.

Source: *Key Facts At a Glance*. Bureau of Justice Statistics. http://bjs.ojp.usdoj.gov. Accessed March 15, 2010.

offenders have not been studied. One can make the argument that because female offenders often target children they know, there is no need to search the Internet for victims. The research is certainly more conclusive when it comes to victims. The authors of a 2007 article in the *Journal of Adolescent Health* found that females were more likely than males to receive requests for sexual pictures. Females were 3.69 times more likely to receive online requests for sexual pictures, and females were almost twice as likely as males to receive sexual solicitations in general. Whereas 35 percent of boys received such solicitations, 65 percent of girls received sexual solicitations.

GENDER AND BULLYING

Both boys and girls engage in bullying and cyber-bullying. In a 2008 study in *Deviant Behavior,* the authors did not find any meaningful gender differences in cyber-bullying behaviors; 18 percent of males and 15.6 percent of females engaged in cyber-bullying.

The authors of a 2008 study in the *Scandinavian Journal of Psychology* indicated, however, that boys are more likely to be cyber-bullies than girls. In this study, 36.2 percent of victims indicated it was a boy who was the cyber-bully, while only 12.1 percent of victims indicated a girl was responsible.

The author of an article in a 2006 issue of *School Psychology International* looked solely at gender differences in bullying. The author found that 40.8 percent of male students were bullies compared to 27.8 percent of female students. Male students also were more likely to be victims of bullying—53.7 percent of males versus 44.4 percent of females. Male students were twice as likely to be cyber-bullies—22.3 percent versus 11.6 percent of females. However, approximately 25 percent of both male and female students were victims of cyber-bullying.

Some gender differences exist when looking at victims of online predatory or abusive behavior. Authors of a 2009 article in the *Journal of Educational Administration* found a significant gender difference for victims of cyber-bullying. Whereas only 27.9 percent of victims were male, 72.1 percent of victims were female. That is a large difference.

However, the authors of the 2008 study in *Deviant Behavior* did not find much of a gender difference for cyber-bullying victims. In this case, 32.7 percent of males and 36.4 percent of females were victims of cyber-bullying.

It sometimes can be difficult to estimate gender differences. An article in a 2009 issue of *School Psychology International* indicated that 23 percent of cyber-bullies pretend to be of a different gender.

GENDER AND ONLINE BEHAVIORS

It is important to understand any gender differences that exist for online behavior, because an understanding of these differences may help provide more insight into patterns of victimization. Online information can be used to harass, stalk, bully, or demean users.

The authors of a study in a 2009 issue of *Computers in Human Behavior* examined what personal information is disclosed by users on Facebook. The authors found that males and females generally shared the same amount of information. The one exception the authors found was that males tended to share more about their religious and political views than did females.

In a 2010 study found in *Computers in Human Behaviors,* researchers examined how visual cues influenced friendship patterns on

Facebook. The authors found that males and females were more likely to initiate friendships with the opposite sex if an attractive picture was in the profile. However, men were more likely than women to initiate friendships with the opposite sex if a picture was not present. In other words, men are more likely to "take a chance" on a female who may not be attractive. Women, however, are less willing to take such a chance.

An article in a 2009 issue of *Computers in Human Behavior* focused on risk-taking and privacy concerns. The authors of this article found that women have more privacy concerns than men. Slightly more than 85 percent of men used their real name on their profiles, while 76.3 percent of women did so. Twelve percent of men listed their home address on their profile, compared to only 6.6 percent of women.

Almost 87 percent of women wrote comments on other users' profile pages. Slightly more than 73 percent of men wrote comments on other profiles. Men were much more willing to list their instant messenger information on their profile. More than 61 percent of men listed this information, compared to only 35 percent of women. Men were also more likely than women to list their phone number (14.5 percent versus 3.9 percent). Overall, females are more concerned about privacy than men. Women do not provide as much information as men in their profiles.

See also: Bullies and Cyber-bullying; Internet Safety; Prevalence and Statistics; Sexual Predators, Online; Social Networking Web Sites

FURTHER READING
Kelsey, Todd. *Social Networking Spaces.* New York: Apress, 2010.
Ray, Audacia. *Naked on the Internet: Hookups, Downloads and Cashing In on Internet Sexploration.* Berkeley, Calif.: Seal Press, 2007.
Sandler, Corey. *Living With the Internet and Online Dangers.* New York: Facts On File, 2010.

■ HATE CRIMES AND ONLINE PREDATORS

Internet-facilitated harm intended to hurt or intimidate someone because of his or her race, ethnicity, religion, sexual orientation, or

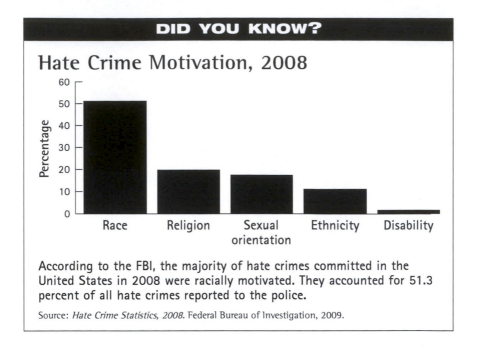

DID YOU KNOW?

Hate Crime Motivation, 2008

According to the FBI, the majority of hate crimes committed in the United States in 2008 were racially motivated. They accounted for 51.3 percent of all hate crimes reported to the police.

Source: *Hate Crime Statistics, 2008.* Federal Bureau of Investigation, 2009.

disability. Online predators encompass more than just adults looking to victimize children. Predators also can include adults or juveniles looking to target members of other groups. Hate crimes are motivated by bias or prejudice toward a specific group.

The Internet has enabled hate groups to spread their messages to a larger population. Hate groups also use social networking Web sites to reach out to people with similar views. Unfortunately, the Internet is an excellent recruiting tool for these groups because the First Amendment protects speech, including hate speech.

HATE CRIME OVERVIEW

Offenders who commit hate crimes target a victim because the victim belongs to a particular group, for example, racial, ethnic, religious, age, gender, or sexual orientation. Hate crimes can be crimes against property or persons. What differentiates a hate crime from other offenses is the offender's motivation. In order for a crime to be classified as a hate crime, the offender must have been motivated by hate or prejudice.

Data published by the FBI in 2009 revealed that an estimated 7,783 hate crimes were committed in 2008. Most crimes are nonviolent in nature. The FBI reported that 32.4 percent of hate crimes involved the destruction or damage of property, as well as vandalism. Another 29.5 percent involved intimidating victims. Simple assaults accounted for 19.4 percent of offenses, while 11.2 percent were aggravated assaults.

The Southern Poverty Law Center identified 932 active hate groups in the United States during 2009. Texas had the most groups with 66, followed by California at 60. States such as North Dakota and Vermont had only one identifiable hate group.

HATE WEB SITES

There are plenty of Web sites promoting hate toward different groups. The Simon Wiesenthal Center in Los Angeles estimates that there are 10,000 hate sites around the world. One such Web site, Stormfront, is said to be one of the most heavily visited Web sites for white supremacy. The Ku Klux Klan (KKK) also maintains Web sites dedicated to their cause. An Internet search for "white supremacy" will return more than 1 million results, with many links to white supremacy groups.

The Council of Conservative Citizens is considered an extremist group that promotes white supremacy. Although the group takes a stance on a variety of political and social issues, they also make clear their white supremacy beliefs. On their Web site they have a page with a statement of principles. They believe that Americans are part of European people. The statement goes on to say, "We also oppose all efforts to mix the races of mankind, to promote non-white races over the European-American people through so-called 'affirmative action' and similar measures, to destroy or denigrate the European-American heritage, including the heritage of the Southern people, and to force the integration of the races."

Unfortunately, hate Web sites allow these groups to reach millions of people, people they would not normally have access to because of geographical boundaries. People around the world now can discuss their similar, often biased, views about different groups.

Hate groups and social networking

Hate groups also have taken to social networking Web sites. These groups use Facebook, MySpace, and YouTube to connect with people and share their message. Social networking sites will disable hate profiles when they are reported. However, that is a difficult task given the popularity of social networking Web sites. Facebook reports that it has more than 400 million active users.

Social networking sites have also been developed that are specifically for extremist groups. For example, the Web site New Saxon bills itself as "An Online Community for Whites by Whites." Whether hate groups have their own Web sites or use social networking Web sites, they are better able to spread their messages to a large audience. It has become very easy to recruit people by staying at home and going online.

Q & A

Question: Do hate crime laws help prevent hate crimes?

Answer: Generally speaking, no. In fact, not all states have hate crime laws. In those states, such as in Wyoming, hate crimes do not legally exist, even when a crime is committed because of hate. Also, states with hate crime laws do not always apply to the same groups.

For example, in Colorado the hate crime laws do not extend to a person's sexual orientation. Connecticut's hate crime laws do apply to sexual orientation. To further complicate matters, it is extremely difficult to prove that a person committed a hate crime. Depending on the evidence, it may be easy to show an offender committed a crime, such as robbery or murder, but prosecutors also have to show the crime was motivated by hate. Unless the offender confesses or evidence is found that shows the specific crime was motivated by hate, it is unlikely that a prosecutor can prove this point. Taken together, hate crime laws do not deter people from committing hate crimes.

In 2008, a woman from Oklahoma was murdered in Louisiana by members of the Ku Klux Klan. This story made headlines around the country because the woman had been recruited by the KKK through MySpace. During the initiation ceremony it is believed the woman changed her mind and wanted to leave. Instead, she was murdered.

HATE SPEECH AND THE INTERNET

One area that has received some attention is hate speech, or online talk intended to hurt or intimidate someone. Hate speech is protected by the First Amendment. Regardless of how inflammatory or repulsive the hate content of speech may be, it is not illegal.

That changes when hate speech is targeted at an individual. The First Amendment does not protect abusive or inflammatory speech when an individual is the target. Such speech can be viewed as a threat to a person's safety. Obviously, responses depend on what exactly is said. Blatant remarks indicating that a person will be harmed is illegal. Further, depending on what is said, a person or group can be sued for libel.

A high-profile case that occurred in 2007 illustrates how hate speech can cross the line. Bill White, a neo-Nazi who founded the American National Socialist Workers Party, was arrested and convicted because of his actions conducted over the Internet. In this case, White both called and sent a threatening e-mail to a person who worked for Citibank. White had hired a private investigator to find where this employee lived and then left a message on her answering machine at home. He also sent an e-mail to her work account where he compared her to a federal judge who worked in Chicago. The mother and husband of this judge, Joan Lefkow, had been murdered. By comparing the Citibank employee to the judge, there was an implicit threat against the employee.

Further, part of White's arrest and conviction focused on his actions against others. It was alleged that he made threats against several other people, including a jury member in a federal trial. He also publicly posted personal information about some of his targets, including telephone numbers and home addresses. In December 2009, a jury convicted him on some counts, but acquitted him on others.

Because hate speech is protected, it is difficult, if not impossible, to take down Web sites filled with hate and rhetoric. As indicated above, only when threats are made toward specific individuals can action be taken. The best way to combat hate is to become more educated and to speak out if you know someone who has been victimized.

See also: Internet Safety; Online Victimization, Examples of; Prejudice and Online Behavior; Social Networking Web Sites

FURTHER READING

Chakraborti, Neil. *Hate Crime: Concepts, Policy, Future Directions.* Devon, U.K.: Willan Publishing, 2010.

Dozier, Rush, Jr. *Why We Hate.* Columbus, Ohio: McGraw-Hill, 2003.

Gerstenfled, Phyllis B. *Hate Crimes: Causes, Controls, and Controversies.* Thousand Oaks, Calif.: Sage Publications, 2010.

■ INSTANT MESSAGING

See: Chat Rooms and Instant Messaging

■ INTERNET SAFETY

Steps to protect online users. Several steps can be taken to help remain safe while using the Internet. Tactics include limiting the amount of personal information one shares, using private browsing features of Web browsers, using antivirus software, reporting harassment to the authorities, and taking precautions when meeting people from the Internet.

SHARING PERSONAL INFORMATION

One of the best ways to stay safe when using the Internet is to keep personal information private. This means do not share it with other people. Giving out usernames and passwords to friends or strangers can be dangerous. Other people can then log in and abuse that information.

It is also important to determine how *much* information to make available to other people. Social networking Web sites allow users to determine how much information they want to share and who is allowed to see it. Authors of an article in a 2008 issue of the *Journal of Adolescence* studied the type of information people place on their MySpace profile. Although 38.4 percent of users included their first name, only 8.8 percent of users included their whole name. People were more relaxed about sharing their location, with 81.2 percent of users naming the city they live in. Authors of a 2009 study in the journal *Computers in Human Behavior* found that 81.8 percent of users used their real name in their profiles. (There was no mention if this included both the first and last name.) Only 9.4 percent said they put their phone number on their profile.

Fact Or Fiction?

People who have friends on Facebook typically do not know each other.

The Facts: It turns out that the overwhelming majority of Facebook users know most or all of their online friends in real life. A 2008 report by the

Internet Safety Technical Task Force found that 50 percent of Facebook users know most of the people they interact with. Another 48 percent said they know all of the people. The remaining 2 percent indicated they knew only a few people or none of the people. However, people still take their privacy seriously. Fifty-one percent of males and 71 percent of females indicated they limit access to their personal information.

Sharing pictures with others is another area that requires caution. It is not recommended that people share pictures that depict potentially embarrassing or illegal behavior. That can come back to haunt a person, both personally and professionally. The authors of a 2008 article in the *Journal of Adolescence* found that 56.9 percent of users included a picture of themselves on their profile. Only 5.4 percent of users included a picture of themselves in either a swimsuit or underwear. An average of four pictures could be found on a profile.

PRIVATE BROWSING

Private browsing is a feature that now can be found in the popular **Web browser** software, such as Firefox, Safari, and Internet Explorer. Private browsing allows the user to access the Internet without collecting any information. For example, a browser keeps track of the Web sites a user visits. This information is kept in the browser's history, allowing people to see what Web sites have been visited. Private browsing does not collect this information. A Google search on private browsing will show that some people refer to this as "porn mode." Such comments are made because men (typically) can go to pornography sites and no one will know about it.

One of the best reasons to use private browsing is that Web sites cannot store cookies on the computer. **Cookies** are bits of information that a Web site uses to personalize a user's visit. According to Mozilla, the company that developed Firefox, cookies can collect personal information, such as an e-mail address, telephone number, name, and address. However, the company goes on to state that the only way this information can be stored in a cookie is if a user provides it in the first place. For example, social networking Web sites require a person to fill out registration information. This information then can be stored in a cookie. Using a private browsing feature prevents this from happening.

Q & A

Question: Should I worry about providing personal information to legitimate companies?

Answer: It is important to keep track of what information you provide to companies. Generally speaking, your information should be safe. However, there are countless instances where a company's secure data was breached. This can cause problems if that data can be accessed for identity theft.

In 2010, Lincoln National Corporation discovered their secure systems *may* have been breached. An unidentified person indicated that a username and password had been distributed among employees. Under company policy this information was not to be shared among employees. This could be used to access personal account information. As a result the accounts for 1.2 million customers may have been compromised.

In another example, personal information of 250,000 people from the Bill Clinton administration and White House visitors was being sent to the National Archives. The hard drive containing the data disappeared. Part of the data included social security numbers.

Unfortunately, no matter how many steps a person takes to try and prevent private information from being stolen, there is always a chance it could happen. As these examples demonstrate, this can happen electronically or by using an old-fashioned method and stealing the equipment with the personal information.

Other benefits of private browsers

Private browsing mode also prevents other information from being saved. Many browsers have an auto-fill or auto-complete feature. This is a time saving feature because users do not have to reenter the same information over and over again. When buying products online, a user needs to enter shipping and billing information. This information can be saved so when a user buys items from the same Web site or other Web sites, the browser will automatically fill in the information. When in private browsing mode, however, this information will not be saved for future use.

Another benefit of private browsing is the passwords will not be saved during the session. Also, if a user allows the browser to automatically fill in password fields when logging on, private browsing prevents this from happening.

More privacy protection

In addition to using private browsing features in Web browsers, people can purchase software that offers privacy protection. This software prevents Web sites from secretly gathering information from your computer. This type of software makes it easier to deal with privacy settings.

There are also Web sites that allow for private browsing. A user can go to such a site and then enter the address of a Web site to visit. The first Web site protects the user, because the second Web site cannot collect a user's information. In a sense, these Web sites run "interference" so that other Web sites cannot see the user. Of course, these Web sites may collect information themselves, thereby defeating the purpose of private browsing.

SECURITY MEASURES

In addition to using private browsing features, there are other security measures users can take. It is critical that people have antivirus software to protect their computers and data.

Kaspersky Lab, a security company that makes antivirus software, produced a report in 2010 on available malware programs. The company recorded more than 33 million pieces of malware. In 2008 and 2009, there were approximately 15 million pieces of malware identified. The number of malware programs has jumped dramatically: Between 1992 and 2007 there were 2 million pieces of malware identified.

Malware can collect personal data and transmit it to another user, one way in which cyber-criminals engage in identity theft. Antivirus programs help protect users' information.

Another security feature that helps protect against computer attacks is a **firewall**. A firewall is a program or hardware device that allows a person to use the Internet while preventing others on the Internet from seeing the user's computer. The firewall inspects all information being sent to and from the computer. Information that should not be transmitted is blocked. What is and is not allowed is determined by the user when configuring the firewall. Firewalls also can learn what information to allow and what to deny. When confronted with information that is questionable, a firewall can ask the user what to do. This gives users control over the flow of data.

REPORT HARASSMENT AND THREATS

Victims of online harassment often do not report what happens. For example, children and teenagers who are bullied rarely let their family or school know what is happening. In a 2008 article in the *Scandinavian Journal of Psychology,* 50 percent of cyber-bully victims did not tell anyone. None of the students reported the incidents to their teachers. Only 8.9 percent told a guardian or parent.

The authors of an article in a 2009 issue of the *Journal of Educational Administration* discovered that only 35.9 percent of cyber-bully victims told their parents. Only 16.7 percent reported the incidents to school officials. Although it will not always be possible to stop cyber-bullying, victims should report their experiences to family and school officials.

MEETING PEOPLE FROM THE INTERNET

It is not advisable to meet someone from the Internet in a private setting. First meetings should take place in public settings. This reduces the chance that something bad can happen. Until people meet in person there is always a chance, regardless of how small it may be, that people are not who they claim to be. Even dating Web sites recommend meeting people for the first time in a public setting. It is also a good idea to let friends or family know when a meeting is going to take place. In the event that something uncomfortable, threatening, or obtrusive does happen, other people will know who you were going to meet and where.

An extreme example of the dangers associated with meeting people from the Internet is the "Craigslist Killer." Philip Markoff, a 24-year-old medical student, was accused of killing a woman he met through the erotic services section of Craigslist. Markoff also had robbed two other women, both of whom he met the same way. Markoff never stood trial for these crimes because he committed suicide in August 2010. This tragedy again illustrates the need for using practical measures when meeting a person from the Internet. Despite the fact that secrecy may have been sought because of the proposed sexual nature of the Markoff encounter, meetings should take place in protected settings.

Children should never meet people from the Internet without a parent being present. Although child abductions are rare, common sense dictates that no child or teenager should meet a stranger for the first time without some form of adult supervision.

See also: Cyber-crimes and Law Enforcement; Online Victimization, Examples of; Phishing and Pharming; Sexual Predators, Online; Social Networking Web Sites

FURTHER READING
Kelsey, Todd. *Social Networking Spaces*. New York: Apress, 2010.
Roddel, Victoria. *The Ultimate Guide to Internet Safety*. Raleigh, N.C.:
  Lulu.com, 2009.

■ LAWS AGAINST INTERNET PREDATORS

Legislation to protect children from online offenders. Laws exist at the state and federal level that are designed specifically to protect children from harmful material found on the Internet. The laws focus on restricting access to inappropriate Web sites, such as chat rooms, pornographic sites, or other sites deemed harmful. These laws only apply to schools and libraries that receive public funding for Internet services. Several laws have been invalidated because they were ruled unconstitutional for infringing on free speech. Laws must be written in a manner that protects minors from harmful Web sites while still allowing adults access to such Web sites.

CHILDREN'S ONLINE PRIVACY PROTECTION ACT OF 1998

The Children's Online Privacy Protection Act (COPPA) of 1998 is one of the first laws specifically designed to protect children from possible online dangers. The law was passed to regulate the collection and use of personal information from children. As the Federal Trade Commission (FTC) states

> COPPA requires operators of Web sites directed to children under 13 years old that collect personal information from them—and operators of general audience Web sites that knowingly collect personal information from children under 13—to notify parents and obtain their consent before collecting, using, or disclosing any such information. One requirement of the COPPA rule is that Web site operators post a privacy policy that is clear, understandable, and complete.

The FTC, which is responsible for enforcing this law, has discovered numerous companies that have not been in compliance with the law. In 2003, the FTC fined two companies—Mrs. Field's Cookies and Hershey Foods Corporation—for violating the law. At the time, these two companies received some of the largest fines associated with breaking this law. Mrs. Field's Cookies was fined $100,000, because they collected private information from children without obtaining parental consent. Hershey was fined $85,000. The company stated that children needed to have parents fill out an online parental consent form before children could provide any information. The problem was that there were no safeguards to ensure that parents actually provided their consent.

Unlike other laws discussed in this section, COPPA has not been challenged in court. The law focuses on privacy rights and does not deal with freedom of speech issues. The law is still in effect, and many companies still receive fines because they are inappropriately collecting data from children. For example, in 2009, a company called the Iconix Brand Group was fined $250,000 for violating this law. In particular, Iconix required consumers on several of its brand-specific Web sites to provide personal information if they wanted to receive updates or enter contests. The information included full name, e-mail address, ZIP code, and in some cases, mailing address, gender, and telephone number.

TEENS SPEAK

I Enjoy Hassle-Free Internet Use

My friends think it is so cool to view porn on the Internet. Apparently they feel like they're more grownup or something. Personally I think the stuff is gross. As it is, I'm exposed to more than enough of it when I'm at home surfing on the Web. Even with the pop-up blockers and some parental supervision software my parents have, some of that stuff still gets through.

When I'm at school I don't have to worry about it. There are a lot of Web sites we can't access. I haven't seen any gross sex pictures at school. The only thing I hate is that we can't chat online. I usually finish my computer lab assignments quickly and then sit around bored. It would be cool if I could chat with some friends around the country. But that's not allowed, and if I want to do it I have to try and use my cell phone to send messages. If we get caught, our phones are confiscated and we get hit with a week's worth of detention. Even though I'm glad the school takes steps to protect us from pornography, sometimes I think they take it too far. It's my phone—if I want to text other people in my free time, I should be able to.

CHILD ONLINE PROTECTION ACT

The Child Online Protection Act (COPA) was passed by Congress in 1998. The purpose of the law was to help restrict access by minors to content that was considered "harmful." Although the law was passed, it was never enforced. A court issued an injunction against enforcing the law. In 2004, the U.S. Supreme Court declared the law to be unconstitutional. The Court indicated that the law was too restrictive, thereby violating the free speech clause in the First Amendment.

CHILDREN'S INTERNET PROTECTION ACT

The Children's Internet Protection Act was passed in 2000 and took effect on April 1, 2001. The law was passed to help address concerns about children having access to offensive material on the Internet. The law only applies to schools and libraries that receive funding for communications technology, such as the Internet.

There are several requirements of the law. Schools and libraries receiving the federal funding must certify that they have Internet safety policies that include technology protection measures. According to the FCC, these protection measures must block or filter Internet access to pictures that are obscene, to child pornography, or to images harmful to minors. Schools and libraries adopting these measures must provide notice and hold at least one public hearing about the proposal.

Schools must adopt and enforce a policy to monitor the online activities of minors. Both schools and libraries are required to adopt and implement an Internet safety policy that addresses

- access by minors to inappropriate materials on the Internet
- safety and security of minors when using forms of direct electronic communications such as e-mail and chat rooms
- unauthorized access and other illegal activities by minors online; unauthorized disclosure, use, and dissemination of personal information about minors
- measures restricting minors' access to materials harmful to them

DELETING ONLINE PREDATORS ACT

The Deleting Online Predators Act of 2006 was another attempt to pass a law protecting children from online predators. The Act was passed by the U.S. House of Representatives and sent to a committee in the Senate. However, the committee never considered the bill, effectively killing it.

In 2007, the Deleting Online Predators Act was once again introduced by the House. However, this time the bill never made it out of a House committee, again killing it.

There were only a couple of key features in the act. First, schools and libraries would have to monitor the online activities of minors. This would be done by blocking Web sites that have materials that are considered "obscene," "child pornography," or "harmful to minors." Schools would have to block access to commercial social networking Web sites and chat rooms. The only exception would be online use for educational purposes, such as research, and there would need to be adult supervision.

Public libraries would need parental consent for minors to access social networking Web sites and chat rooms. Libraries would also have to inform parents about the possibility that sexual predators use these Web sites to target children.

PROBLEMS WITH PROTECTION LAWS

If the bill is ever introduced again and becomes law, there no doubt will be a host of lawsuits from civil rights organizations. Because the act prohibits access to certain Web sites, it is viewed as infringing on First Amendment rights. In particular, it is seen as **censoring** content, which is a violation of the First Amendment.

Similar challenges have been made against the Children Internet Protection Act. This was legislation that became law in 2000. The goal of the act was to filter offensive online materials in schools and libraries. Only schools and libraries that received funding for Internet access would have to comply with the law. Further, if an adult wanted to access filtered content for research or lawful purposes, the filtering software would be temporarily disabled on that computer.

There is a fundamental problem with any legislation that tries to filter online content, because such restrictions, opponents say, infringe on free speech. Further, it is argued that once the government begins censoring some material, where will it end? This is known as the **slippery slope argument.** Essentially, once people can censor

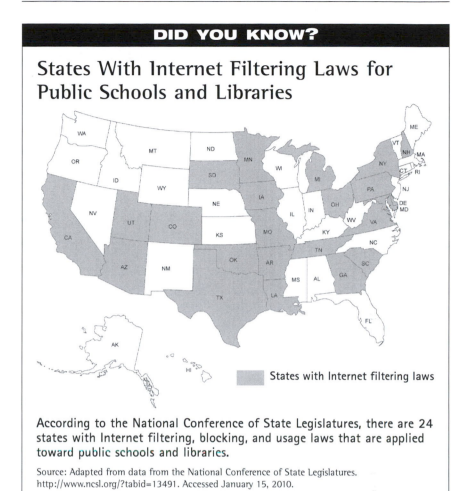

DID YOU KNOW?

States With Internet Filtering Laws for Public Schools and Libraries

States with Internet filtering laws

According to the National Conference of State Legislatures, there are 24 states with Internet filtering, blocking, and usage laws that are applied toward public schools and libraries.

Source: Adapted from data from the National Conference of State Legislatures. http://www.ncsl.org/?tabid=13491. Accessed January 15, 2010.

some material, they may believe it is okay to censor more and more material. The question becomes, where does the censorship end? The answer is simple: Do not let censorship start and then society will not have to worry about a slippery slope effect.

However, the situation becomes more complicated when minors are involved. Minors are prohibited from being exposed to certain materials, such as pornography. Laws designed to protect minors from such material must be written in a way that they do not also infringe on an adult's right to view that same material. This is why laws such as the Child Online Protection Act are declared illegal or unconstitutional.

ELECTRONIC SECURITY AND TARGETING OF ONLINE PREDATORS ACT

In 2008, New York State passed the Electronic Security and Targeting of Online Predators Act (E-STOP). The law requires sexual offenders to register their Internet accounts and screen names with law enforcement. Social networking Web sites then can access this information to prevent sex offenders from using their services. The law also prevents "dangerous" sex offenders from using the Internet to communicate with minors or access pornography. Registered offenders who fail to report their Internet accounts to law enforcement can be charged with a felony.

The problem with this legislation is enforcement. At the end of 2008, there were 28,017 sex offenders registered in New York. Proactively investigating which offenders have Internet access and social networking accounts is impossible. Relying on registered sex offenders to be completely honest is also unrealistic. Although the law is supposed to help protect children from online predators, by design it is not very effective. If anything, it allows prosecutors to file additional charges against a predator who is caught using the Internet to find children (assuming the predator did not register his screen names).

The law has helped Facebook and MySpace identify some online predators. According to the New York attorney general's office, by December 2009 Facebook had disabled 2,782 accounts linked to registered sex offenders. MySpace had disabled 1,796 accounts.

INTERNET STOPPING ADULTS FACILITATING THE EXPLOITATION OF TODAY'S YOUTH (SAFETY) ACT OF 2009

Another federal act that still lingers in a congressional committee is the Internet Stopping Adults Facilitating the Exploitation of Today's Youth (SAFETY) Act. This is *not* an act designed to help protect youth from Internet predators. Instead, the act acknowledges the potential dangers of Internet predators and authorizes grant funding to conduct more research on the subject.

Some of the areas in which the act calls for research include online activities of sex offenders, minor-to-minor online solicitation, use of digital media (pictures, videos) and how that influences harassment, and the creation of problematic content by youth. It is hoped that this research can then identify best practices for Internet safety and education.

See also: Bullies and Cyber-bullying; Hate Crimes and Online Predators; Online Predators, Characteristics of; Privacy Issues; Sexual Predators, Online

FURTHER READING
Rustad, Michael L. *Internet Law in a Nutshell.* Eagan, Minn.: West Group, 2009.

■ MEDIA AND ONLINE PREDATORS, THE
Media coverage of those who victimize others online. The media plays an important role in society by providing the public with news. However, news organizations have to compete against other companies, and many are going out of business. These organizations need to find ways to attract viewers or readers. As a result, the media tend to focus on sensational topics, such as violent crimes and online predator behavior.

There is no authoritative published research on the media's coverage of online predators. However, NBC devoted numerous episodes of *Dateline NBC* to online predators in the To Catch a Predator series, which attracted millions of viewers until controversy ended the show in 2007.

THE GOAL OF NEWS ORGANIZATIONS
Most people think the media's goal is to provide news coverage. However, the goal of organizations is to make a profit. The newspaper industry, for example, has been financially devastated as more and more people get their news from the Internet. In 2009, the *Seattle-Post Intelligencer* stopped publication and went to a stripped-down online version. The newspaper had existed for 146 years. The *Rocky Mountain News* in Colorado shut down two months before its 150th year of operation. Those newspaper organizations that have stayed in business have scaled down to help break even financially or maintain a profit.

Broadcast companies also have been hurt because of loss of advertising revenue. Disputes between companies and cable carriers have repeatedly popped up. For example, in 2010 there was a dispute between ABC and Cablevision over revenue. ABC wanted more money, while Cablevision did not want to pay more for providing ABC channels to its viewers. On March 7, 2010, ABC stopped broadcasting its service to Cablevision's customers in the New York City area. This was a significant move, because the Academy Awards were being broadcast on ABC that night. As a result, Cablevision customers were angry and had to try and find other ways to watch this popular show, until some deal was negotiated late that evening.

The point is that media companies need to make money to stay in business. This means that news programs have to find ways to attract viewers. It is no longer good enough simply to report on news stories. The stories need to grab viewers' attention and be better than the stories found on competing news programs. Organizations have to decide which stories to report, what angle or hook to use to grab viewers, what to say, and how to say it.

DECISIONS IN MEDIA COVERAGE

To date, no studies have been conducted of media coverage of online predators. It is not possible to determine the accuracy of media reports about Internet predators. It is also impossible to determine how many stories cover the same incident. As mentioned above, stories that will grab the public's interest will command the most media attention. The well-being of children is always of interest to the public. Violent crime and safety is a public concern. Taken together, stories that deal with children being seduced or abducted by strangers they meet on the Internet will command attention, and these are the stories the media will report.

Q & A

Question: If the media reports or publishes stories about crime, doesn't that mean the stories are important?

Answer: Crime and safety are important topics in society. There's no question about that. The problem is the accuracy of the stories that are reported. According to a 2009 report by the Bureau of Justice Statistics, there were more than 16 million property crimes and slightly more than 4.8 million violent crimes in the United States during 2008. However, media reports focus on violent crimes, even though these make up fewer than 25 percent of all crimes.

A 2010 report from the University of Southern California found that 33 percent of news broadcasts in Los Angeles started with crime stories. According to the authors, about half of those stories dealt with "murder, robbery, assault, kidnapping, property crime, traffic crime, and other common crime." The authors also noted that 25 percent of the stories focused on crimes that were not local to the Los Angeles media market. Even though crime and safety are important issues, the media prefer to capitalize on sensational crimes that will grab a person's attention and hopefully keep it for the remainder of the news broadcast.

A 2008 study in the online journal *First Monday* did provide some evidence of the increased attention the media has paid to online predators. The author found that three stories about online predators appeared in major newspapers across the United States during 2000. In 2007, there were 457 stories about online predators. *That is a 1,500 percent increase in seven years.* The author also noted that during the first two months of 2008, 110 stories had already been published about online predators.

To Catch a Predator

Dateline NBC is a television news-magazine show that is broadcast on NBC. The program does investigative stories on topics that are of interest to the public. From 2004 through 2007, there were several episodes devoted to Internet predators. *To Catch a Predator* became a series, with approximately 12 episodes airing during the three-year period.

The premise of the show was simple—lure Internet predators to a house where they believed they would have sex with a child or teenager. Adults would pose as children on the Internet and chat with adults looking for sex. Transcripts of the conversations would show that the suspect believed he was talking with a minor. The undercover adult would make it clear he was a minor. At some point a meeting would be proposed and the "child" would invite the offender to her house. When the suspect would arrive, the show's host would confront the suspect about his actions. This was all caught on camera.

At first the show's producers did not work with law enforcement. After a couple of episodes, however, the show started working with police. The police would arrest those offenders who showed up at the house looking for sex with minors. The arrests would take place after the show's host interviewed suspects about their actions. The show also started working with the online group Perverted Justice. This group is dedicated to reducing online predatory behavior and helping catch predators. The organization is still in existence and works with law enforcement to help catch online predators.

To Catch a Predator stopped airing in 2007. Repeats occasionally air on cable, and episodes also can be found online. The show was criticized by many for taking journalism too far. The goal of journalists is to report stories, not create them. By setting up sting operations with police and working with Perverted Justice, critics felt the producers of the show crossed the line.

TV shows as public service?

Regardless of whether the show violated the principles of good journalism, there are some who believe the show provided a public service. Removing these predators from the streets was seen as a victory for child protection. Unfortunately, this did not happen. The *New York Times* published a story on the show on August 17, 2007. They noted that 256 men had been arrested in the various sting operations. Fewer than half of them were convicted of a crime.

There also were claims that the show was less than honest in its approach to catching predators. One of the show's producers, Marsha Bartel, alleged she had been fired when she said the show violated the ethics of journalism. Bartel filed a lawsuit against NBC, which was ultimately dismissed. Bartel claimed that NBC had paid officers to participate in stings so more drama could unfold on camera. It also was discovered that Perverted Justice was paid a consulting fee for each episode on which they helped. Depending on the source of information, the payments ranged from $70,000 to $150,000 per episode. Critics argued that this created a conflict of interest, as Perverted Justice was directly involved in the process of luring offenders and then profiting from their activities.

In Bartel's lawsuit, she indicated that Perverted Justice did not always provide full transcripts of chat sessions. Therefore, it was not possible to verify the accuracy of the chat sessions when suspects were confronted. This also contributed to cases not being prosecuted after a suspect was arrested. In one instance, a district attorney did not prosecute 23 individuals who were arrested as part of a sting operation. The prosecutor indicated that Perverted Justice did not provide enough evidence that could be used against suspects.

Predators are not everywhere

Regardless of any ethical or legal problems associated with sting operations by *To Catch a Predator,* the show helped to create an unrealistic fear about Internet predators. There are predators on the

Internet who are willing to seek and meet children for sex. Obviously children, teens, and parents need to be aware of this possibility and act in a responsible manner. However, when a TV show airs with suspect after suspect being arrested, it contributes to an unrealistic image that these offenders are everywhere, just waiting for the opportunity to pounce.

Q & A

Question: Are child abductions common?

Answer: Child abductions are not very common. According to the National Center for Missing and Exploited Children, there were 194 AMBER Alerts during 2008. AMBER alerts are issued when a child under the age of 18 has been abducted. Once law enforcement confirms an abduction, believes the child is in serious danger, and has enough information to release, the alert will be issued. In 100 of these cases, the abductor was a family member. In 70 cases, the abductor was someone unknown to the child or family. Twenty-one instances were deemed as the child's being lost or missing, with no information as to why the child was missing.

Other data also indicates that child abductions are rare. During 2008, 13,933 children were reported missing to the police. Only 18 cases were reported as kidnappings, while 31 cases were classified as a family abduction. In 2008, there were 114,157 children reported missing in the state of California. Thirty-five cases were classified as a child being abducted by a stranger or nonfamily member. Family abductions accounted for another 1,363 reports. In 417 cases the reports were classified as "suspicious circumstances," which means a stranger abduction may have occurred. Overall, child abductions are rare events; being abducted by a stranger is even less common.

MEDIA COVERAGE AND ARRESTS OF PREDATORS

Predators always attempt to meet children or teens in person. In the TV series, that was easy to accomplish because the suspect was given the "child's" address. A 2009 report by the Crimes Against Children Research Center provides data that shows there will be a significant jump in arrests when a suspect is told where to meet the "child." Between 2000 and 2006, there was a 381 percent increase in the number of arrests made against predators looking to meet children or teens. In 2000, there were 664 such arrests. In 2006, the number of arrests went up to 3,100. During the same period, there was only a 21 percent increase in arrests where a predator came into contact with a real victim. In 2000, police arrested 508 suspects. In 2006, there were 615 such arrests.

See also: Online Predators, Characteristics of; Online Victimization, Examples of; Prevalence and Statistics; Sexual Predators, Online

FURTHER READING
Carrabine, Eamonn. *Crime, Culture, and the Media.* Boston: Polity, 2008.
Censer, Jack R. *On the Trial of the D.C. Sniper: Fear and the Media.* Charlottesville: University of Virginia Press, 2010.
Fuhrman, Mark. *The Murder Business: How the Media Turns Crime Into Entertainment and Subverts Justice.* Washington, D.C.: Regnery Publishing, 2009.

■ MYSPACE
See: Prevalence and Statistics; Social Networking Web Sites

■ ONLINE PREDATORS, CHARACTERISTICS OF
Common traits of those who seek to victimize someone else by abusing or demeaning that person online. Online predators are predominantly male, older, with many being in relationships and employed. Offenders are not typically impulsive, have self-esteem issues, and experience difficulties in relating to others.

DEMOGRAPHIC CHARACTERISTICS
Nearly 100 percent of online predators are male. According to the Geneva, Illinois, police department, if a woman is involved, it is usually as an accomplice to a male predator. Online predators tend to be at least 35 years old. They are typically married or have been married.

A 2005 study in *Swiss Medical Weekly* provided demographic information on offenders convicted of purchasing child pornography on the Internet. All offenders were male and their average age was

39.8 years. One-third were never married or had been intimately involved with a woman. The remaining two-thirds were currently married, involved in a relationship, or divorced.

A 2007 study in *Psychology, Crime & Law* produced similar findings. The average age of the offenders was almost 41 years. The sample consisted of all males. Slightly more than 73 percent of the men were employed, with 36.7 percent in professional occupations. Another 10 percent held information technology (IT) positions. Thirty percent were married, and another 16.7 percent were in relationships.

Q & A

Question: How do online predators make contact with children and teens?

Answer: A 2007 report in the *Journal of Child Sexual Abuse* provides insight into the methods online predators use to connect with children and teens. The authors found that 81 percent of offenders visited chat rooms for minors. Almost 50 percent also indicated that they reviewed online profiles of minors. Another strategy was to view the screen names. If a name indicated a person's age or referenced sex in any manner, the offender would target that person. Twenty-nine percent of offenders pretended they were children when talking with other children and teens. Once contact was made, 97 percent of the offenders indicated they would engage in sexual conversations.

PSYCHOLOGICAL CHARACTERISTICS

Online predators are generally not thought of as pedophiles. The American Psychiatric Association defines a pedophile as someone who is sexually attracted to prepubescent children, those younger than about 12. Young children may have access to the Internet, however, they don't usually knew about social networking and chat rooms. As a result, online predators have limited access to young children. However, online predators *are* considered child molesters because they target adolescents.

The authors of a 2008 article in the journal *American Psychologist* reviewed evidence on the characteristics of online child molesters. One trait of online child molesters is the lack of violence. These predators have the self-control needed to develop relationships with adolescents over time. This is consistent with findings from a 2008 article in the *Journal of Nervous and Mental Disease*. In that article, the authors examined personality trait differences among pedophiles, opiate addicts, and healthy volunteers. The authors found that pedophiles had levels of self-control similar to healthy volunteers.

A 2002 study in *Comprehensive Psychiatry* also yielded similar results. Male pedophiles did not display higher levels of impulsiveness when compared to healthy volunteers.

Whatever means predators use to lure victims, the evidence suggests they do not act impulsively. This is part of the reason why they can be potentially so dangerous: they act rationally and plan things out.

ONLINE CHILD MOLESTERS AND PORNOGRAPHY

The authors also point out that approximately 40 percent of online child molesters possess child pornography. Because the Internet allows easy access to distribute and collect pornography, many online predators collect it. Further, many predators produce it. The authors indicate that approximately 20 percent of online child molesters took suggestive or explicit photographs of their victims. Predators also convince victims to take pictures of themselves.

TYPES OF ONLINE PREDATORS

The author of an article in a 2007 issue of *Mayo Clinic Proceedings* reviewed material on categorizing online pedophiles. Citing other works, the author found that there are five categories of online pedophiles

- stalkers
- cruisers
- masturbators
- networkers/swappers
- combinations of the other categories

Stalkers are the most dangerous pedophiles, because they use the Internet to gain physical access to children. Cruisers and masturbators rely on the Internet to obtain sexual gratification. Cruisers use chat rooms to engage in **cybersex,** while masturbators view child pornography. Networkers or swappers exchange material over the Internet, such as information and pictures. In very rare cases where children have been abducted by online predators, networkers may arrange to swap children.

The author of the 2007 article in *Mayo Clinic Proceedings* also notes that pedophiles feel inferior, have low self-esteem and emotional immaturity, and internal **dysphoria**. Although these characteristics were applied to pedophiles in general, they can be used for online predators as well.

Fact Or Fiction?

Social networking sites increase the risk of victimization by online predators.

The Facts: The authors of a 2008 article in *American Psychologist* addressed this question. Based on data and interviews they conducted with law enforcement officers, the answer is no. Some cases in 2006 generated a great deal of media attention, which led people to believe this is a widespread problem. Evidence indicates that, while offenders can use social networking sites to try and find potential victims, kids and teenagers are more likely to receive sexual solicitations in chat rooms or through instant messages.

INTERNET PREDATORS AND (CONTACT) CHILD MOLESTERS

Authors of a 2007 study in *Sex Abuse* compared the characteristics of Internet child pornography offenders and child molesters. The authors gathered data from probation and treatment records of convicted sex offenders. Several interesting findings emerged from this information. The Internet offenders had an average of 16,698 images on their computers. However, this number is misleading, as the number ranged from a low of two images to a high of 921,000 images. The large number skews the results.

Another indicator found that Internet offenders had an average of 317.5 pictures on their computers. Sixty-two percent of offenders used search engines to locate the images. Most offenders had a diverse set of pictures. Seventy-one percent had pictures of erotic poses, while 77 percent had pictures of sexual activity. Sadly, 80 percent of offenders had pictures of children being touched in a sexual manner by an adult. Finally, 76 percent of offenders had pictures showing adults performing sexual acts on children.

In contrast to some other studies, the authors found that Internet offenders were younger than child molesters. Internet offenders also were more likely than child molesters to have had prior contact with mental health services. Interestingly, these offenders were also less likely to be in an intimate relationship and live with that person.

OTHER PSYCHOLOGICAL ISSUES

Another psychological aspect of online predators is the use of cognitive distortions, thought patterns that can legitimize unacceptable behavior. In other words, predators find ways to justify their behavior by distorting the acceptability of the behavior and the harm it causes.

Authors of a 2007 study in *Psychology, Crime & Law* examined the cognitive distortions used by Internet and contact offenders. The Internet offenders, who had been convicted of online pornography offenses, felt that children were willing to engage in sex with adults. Surprisingly, the Internet offenders had stronger belief of this distortion than those offenders who actually made contact with children. Internet offenders were also more likely than contact offenders to believe that children can make up their minds about having sex with adults. In a similar vein, in another distorted view, Internet offenders also were more likely to feel that some children are willing and eager to be involved in sexual activities with an adult.

The authors of a 2009 article in *Sexual Abuse: A Journal of Research and Treatment* examined the psychological profile of online sexual offenders and compared it to the profile of contact offenders. Compared to contact offenders, Internet offenders are less likely to engage in cognitive distortions, have a lower level of emotional congruence with children, and are less likely to make quick decisions. However, the findings also indicated that Internet offenders were more likely to identify with fictional characters.

Another study in a 2007 issue of *Psychology, Crime & Law* focused on personality issues of Internet sex offenders. The authors found that a significant portion of the offenders in the study had interpersonal difficulties. In other words, it was difficult for these offenders to interact with other people. That is not surprising since 60 percent of the offenders either had not had a sexual relationship with another adult or had not been able to live with a sexual partner for an extended period of time (at least two years).

The authors also noted that the offenders lacked empathy in relationships and did not value close or lasting relationships. The data also suggested that offenders tend to be withdrawn and feel misunderstood by others. Offenders also tend to be depressed. Seventy-three percent of offenders met the criteria for depression, while another 9 percent experienced dysphoria, an emotional state marked by anxiety, restlessness, and depression. Educating oneself about some of the characteristics can help users avoid them.

See also: Chat Rooms and Instant Messaging; Internet Safety; Media and Online Predators; Pornography and Online Predators; Screen Names; Sexual Predators, Online

FURTHER READING

Salter, Anna. *Predators: Pedophiles, Rapists, and Other Sex Offenders.* Jackson, Tenn.: Basic Books, 2004.
Sax, Robin. *Predators and Child Molesters: What Every Parent Needs to Know to Keep Kids Safe.* Amherst, N.Y.: Prometheus Books, 2009.
Sullivan, Mike. *Online Predators.* Longwood, Fla.: Xulon Press, 2008.

▨ ONLINE VICTIMIZATION, EXAMPLES OF

Ways of demeaning or abusing someone online. There are several types of online victimization, including cyber-bullying, identity theft, harassment, threats, solicitation, and computer threats. Identity theft can be the most serious form of online victimization, as it can take victims years to recover. Children and teenagers can be subjected to cyber-bullying, which is often an extension of regular bullying, the repeated attack by a more powerful person on a less powerful one. Although there is widespread concern about online victimization, fortunately only a fraction of children and teenagers are solicited or harassed.

BULLYING

People can be bullied in person or online. Cyber-bullying is a form of harassment through the Internet. It can occur in e-mails, chat rooms, instant messaging, public forums, and so forth. The goal of cyber-bullying is the same as traditional bullying—to demean a person through ridicule.

Authors of a 2008 study in the *Journal of School Health* found that insults tend to be the most common form of cyber-bullying.

Threats, stealing passwords, and sharing private information and embarrassing pictures are also forms of cyber-bullying. Authors of an article in a 2009 issue of *New Media & Society* surveyed almost 1,100 students between the ages of 10 and 18 years old. Slightly more than 11 percent of the students said they had been victims of cyber-bullying. Eighteen percent admitted to engaging in cyber-bullying. The most common forms of bullying were making insults or threats, pretending to be a victim (deception), and spreading gossip.

IDENTITY THEFT

The most common type of online victimization is attempted and completed identity thefts. In 2009, the FTC received 278,078 complaints about identity theft. This made up 21 percent of all consumer complaints that the FTC received in that year. The FTC learned that 48 percent of people were initially contacted through e-mail.

Phishing and pharming are two methods used to steal information from potential victims for the purposes of identity theft. Phishing involves sending potential victims an e-mail, which typically indicates that the person needs to provide personal information for account verification. Victims are directed to a legitimate-looking Web site that has been designed by the identity thieves. People who follow through with these instructions unknowingly provide financial information to offenders.

Pharming is more dangerous than phishing because e-mail is not used. Attackers target security vulnerabilities of Web sites. When a person goes to a legitimate Web site, he or she is unknowingly redirected to a fraudulent Web site. People then enter personal or account information, thinking they are on the proper Web site.

HARASSMENT, THREATS, AND SOLICITATION

People other than bullies engage in harassment. Strangers can harass users for no apparent reason. Harassment can consist of sending annoying e-mails or instant messages, posting bothersome comments on social Web site pages, writing nasty comments in public forums, and more.

Threats are a more serious form of harassment. Instead of making annoying, but benign, comments, the comments focus on harming a user. Threats can be frightening, especially when they come from a stranger.

Q & A

Question: How often are children and teenagers harassed or solicited over the Internet?

Answer: According to a comprehensive study published in a 2007 issue of the *Journal of Adolescent Health,* 5 percent of children between ages 10 and 12 had received a sexual solicitation. Five percent also had been harassed online. Fifteen percent of teenagers between the ages of 13 and 15 had received sexual solicitations, while 10 percent had been harassed. Teenagers who were 16 or 17 years old were the most likely to be sexually solicited, with 17 percent indicating this happened. Nine percent reported being harassed.

Another form of online victimization is sexual solicitation. This includes being approached by e-mail, instant messaging, in chat rooms, or on public forums for sex or sexual pictures. The author of a 2007 study in the *Journal of Child Sexual Abuse* studied how sex offenders identified and contacted minors over the Internet. Eighty-one percent of the offenders used chat rooms to find potential victims. Almost 49 percent of offenders reviewed online profiles. Another 9.7 percent screened bulletin board postings. Offenders would look at screen names and comments of users. Screen names with sexual references or those that indicated the person was young would attract attention. Fifty-two percent of offenders, after having made contact, would send pictures of child pornography to the kids they spoke with. Ninety-seven percent had explicitly sexual online conversations with the minors they wanted to meet.

Another approach that predators use is **grooming**. This approach tends to be more subtle. Instead of making solicitations immediately, a predator may make the occasional comment about sex. Then the comments and questions increase in frequency. After a while the predator may ask for a picture or send one to the child. The goal is to convince the child that there is nothing wrong with explicit conversations or sharing sexual pictures.

COMPUTER THREATS

Computers can be damaged through the Internet. There are millions of viruses and spyware online. Without the proper security preventions, it is very easy for a computer to become infected with multiple viruses and spyware.

The company Kaspersky, which makes antivirus software, identified approximately 15 million different pieces of malicious programming, such as viruses, in 2009 alone. They have a database containing approximately 34 million pieces of malware that have been discovered since 2003.

Q & A

Question: What are bots?

Answer: Bots stands for Internet robots. These are software applications that automate tasks over the Internet. They perform tasks quickly, whereas it would take a person a great deal of time to accomplish. For example, a bot can send out hundreds or thousands of e-mails in a short period of time. It would take a person hours, days, or weeks to perform the same task. Bots are an important part of spam and viruses. In order to help spread viruses and spam quickly, while reducing the chances of being caught, computer programmers design bots to do the job for them. Bots can collect or harvest information, such as e-mail addresses, and then use that information to spread viruses and spam.

Although malware cannot physically damage a computer, it can cause a user to lose all data. Viruses can corrupt a computer, requiring someone to completely erase the hard drive and reinstall everything. Further, depending on the virus, any backup copies of data may also be infected or corrupted. Although a computer's operating system can be reinstalled, along with the software a user has purchased, it can be costly and time-consuming.

The best way to help prevent this type of problem is to run antivirus and anti-spyware software. Some software packages take care of both issues, while others may only focus on viruses or spyware. Anyone who uses the Internet should have these protections in place.

See also: Bullies and Cyber-bullying; Hate Crimes and Online Predators; Phishing and Pharming; Physical Threats; Sexual Predators, Online

FURTHER READING
Milhorn, H. Thomas. *Cybercrime: How to Avoid Becoming a Victim.* Boca Raton, Fla.: Universal Publishers, 2007.

Palfrey, John, Danah Boyd, and Dena Sacco. *Enhancing Child Safety and Online Technologies: Final Report of the Internet Safety Technical Task Force.* Durham, N.C.: Carolina Academic Press, 2010.

Wall, David S. *Cybercrime: The Transformation of Crime in the Information Age.* Boston: Polity, 2007.

▓ PARENTAL CONTROL

Parental strategies to control children's online behaviors. Several methods can be effective in controlling behavior in an effort to protect one's children or teens. These include talking about Internet dangers, limiting the amount of time spent on the Internet, and installing filtering/monitoring software. Although parents generally tend to express concerns about Internet safety, research indicates that most parents do not place controls on their children's behavior.

CONTROL STRATEGIES

With the Internet and cell phones, it is much easier to connect with other people than in the past. This means it is easier to come into contact with strangers who may or may not have malicious intentions. Concerns about online predators and the potential for abusive behavior over the Internet have many parents worried. The fear of the unknown leads to worries.

There are several steps that parents can use to control their children's online activities. The first approach is to prohibit Internet access from home. However, because that is extreme, one of the best things parents can do is talk to their children about being responsible. Parents should set ground rules, such as not sharing private information. They should acknowledge the potential dangers of the Internet, such as coming into contact with predators or being the victim of identity theft.

Another way to help control behavior is to prohibit Internet access from private bedrooms. Having children use the computer in a common area allows parents and others to monitor behavior. People are less likely to engage in problem behaviors when their parents can see what is going on in a moment's notice. Parents also can limit the amount of time their children spend on the Internet. It may be limited to a specific amount of time or limited to spending time strictly on homework assignments.

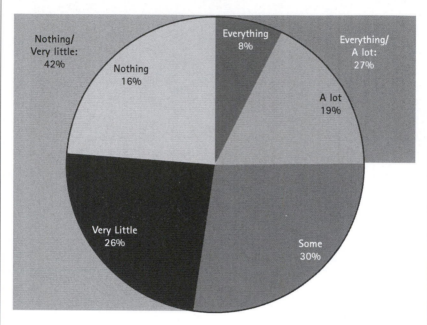

DID YOU KNOW?

How Much Parents Know About Their Teens' Online Activities

Nothing/
Very little:
42%

Nothing
16%

Everything
8%

Everything/
A lot:
27%

A lot
19%

Very Little
26%

Some
30%

Almost half of teenagers surveyed indicated their parents know nothing or very little about their online activities. Only 19 percent of parents, according to teens, know a lot about what their teenagers do online.

Source: *Teen Online and Wireless Safety Survey.* Cox Communications, 2009.

Filtering and monitoring software

Parents also can monitor or control Internet use through software, specific programs that can be used to control what can be done on a computer. This allows parents to monitor what goes on without having to be physically present to do it.

There are numerous software packages available for parents to use. Two of the more popular programs are Net Nanny and Safe Eyes. Net Nanny offers parents several features that can shield children from problematic material and online behavior. For example, profanity is blocked and replaced with symbols such as !, $, &, and *. Pornographic material and Web sites also can be blocked, and parents can specify specific Web sites they wish to block—including gaming, social networking, and other sites. The software also provides instant alerts to cell phones when children are trying to access restricted Web sites.

The Safe Eyes software offers similar controls over Internet use, providing alerts and reports on Internet behavior. Parents can literally see everything their children did while online. The software also can restrict the amount of time a user is on the computer as well as record instant messaging conversations. If children are being harassed or sexually solicited, the parents will know about it.

These are just some of the features found in two filtering programs. Generally speaking, such programs allow parents to both monitor and control online activity. Certainly, however, there are ways to bypass

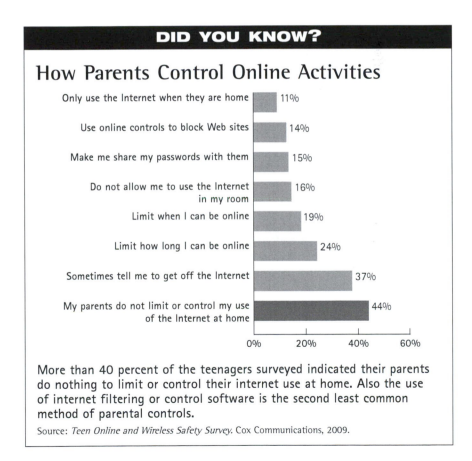

DID YOU KNOW?

How Parents Control Online Activities

Only use the Internet when they are home	11%
Use online controls to block Web sites	14%
Make me share my passwords with them	15%
Do not allow me to use the Internet in my room	16%
Limit when I can be online	19%
Limit how long I can be online	24%
Sometimes tell me to get off the Internet	37%
My parents do not limit or control my use of the Internet at home	44%

More than 40 percent of the teenagers surveyed indicated their parents do nothing to limit or control their internet use at home. Also the use of internet filtering or control software is the second least common method of parental controls.

Source: *Teen Online and Wireless Safety Survey.* Cox Communications, 2009.

these controls. Teenagers will go to the library or a friend's house and use the Internet, and teens who are very knowledgeable about computers can try and deactivate the software. A good safeguard is for parents to talk to their children about potential dangers.

RESEARCH EVIDENCE

Although parents have concerns about their children's safety while using the Internet, there is only a limited amount of research that examines parental perceptions and control strategies. The authors of an article in a 2008 issue of the *Journal of Applied Developmental Psychology* studied the awareness and concerns of parents whose children use MySpace. The authors found that 38 percent of parents had never seen their teenager's MySpace page, with another 14 percent indicating they had almost never seen the page. Only 38 percent of parents ever talked with their teenagers about MySpace, and 40 percent never viewed the pictures their teenagers posted. Ironically, 63 percent of parents believed there are "quite a few" sexual predators found on the Web site. Even though this appears to be a concern of parents, the evidence indicates that parents do not take a protective role in their teenagers' MySpace behaviors. Parents did indicate, however, that they placed some limits on their children's use of MySpace. Sixty-one percent of parents with children between the ages of 10 and 13 imposed limits, while only 39 percent with children who were 14 or 15 had placed limits. Parents of teenagers between the ages of 16 and 17 were even less likely to place limits, with only 24 percent of parents doing so.

Use of filtering software

There is not much evidence regarding how frequently parents use filtering software. Authors of a study in a 2006 issue of *Youth & Society* found that 19 percent of teens indicated there was filtering software on their computers. A more recent study in a 2008 issue of the *Journal of Broadcasting & Electronic Media* had similar findings. The authors reported that only 33 percent of parents used filtering software on their children's computers. Twenty-three percent of parents indicated they installed monitoring software on the computers.

Other protective controls

Although there were not many parents who used filtering or monitoring software, many of these parents took other steps to help control online behaviors. Sixty-seven percent of parents did not allow their children to give out personal information. Thirty-four percent of parents stayed nearby while their children were on the Internet, while 46 percent indicated they watched what their children were doing. Thirty percent of parents would check the Web sites their children visited, while 17 percent read their children's e-mails.

SOME CONCLUSIONS

Collectively, the evidence seems to suggest that parents are concerned about their children's online behavior. However, that concern does not often translate into action. Less than 50 percent of the parents in these studies took steps to help prevent problems from arising. Although 67 percent of parents in one study prohibited their children from giving out personal information, there was no mention of how this was enforced. Telling kids not to do something and having them follow through are two different things. Clearly additional research is needed on this subject to better understand what are the best protective steps parents can take and why.

See also: Internet Safety; Online Victimization, Examples of; Phishing and Pharming; Privacy Issues; Social Networking Web Sites

FURTHER READING
Kelsey, Todd. *Social Networking Spaces*. New York: Apress, 2010.
Roddel, Victoria. *The Ultimate Guide to Internet Safety*. Raleigh, N.C.: Lulu.com, 2009.

■ PEERS AND PEER PRESSURE

The strong influence that one's peers have on attitudes and behavior. Peer pressure occurs when friends or people in a person's **reference group** "persuade" that person to do something. Peer pressure influences almost all teenagers. Fear of being disliked and low self-esteem contribute to the success of peer pressure, which influences behavior in both the physical and virtual worlds. Although to date there is little research on peer pressure and online behavior, the research that does exist indicates that peer pressure does influence behaviors associated with social networking and cyber-bullying.

WHAT IS PEER PRESSURE?

Typically, the person being pressured does not want to engage in the behavior. The behavior may be negative, such as shoplifting, smoking, or skipping school. It may also be positive, such as taking responsibility for an action, finishing assignments, or studying for an exam.

Peer pressure works because people are afraid others will not like them if they fail to follow through on these behaviors. It is the fear of what will happen by saying no that helps compel someone to go along with what other people want. This includes fear of being rejected, teased, or liked by others. Most teenagers are not immune to peer pressure. It is rare that someone will do what he or she wants without worrying what others think.

There are certain factors that influence a person's susceptibility to peer pressure. Fear of one's peers or weak ties to friends both play a role; these indicate that, at times, fear of losing so-called friends is more important than doing the right thing. People also do not want their peers to turn on them, thereby being subjected to bullying.

TEENS SPEAK

I Should Have Said No!

I let my friends talk me into doing something really stupid. Several of them were taking pictures while only wearing skimpy underwear. Then they were going to upload them to an adult dating Web site. I didn't think it was the best idea and really didn't want to do it. But they kept harping on me. How "everyone is doing it" and "it'll make you look like a sexy adult." Finally I gave in and let them take pictures of me in my bra and panties. We created some online profiles and included the pictures. Unfortunately, a couple of weeks later another guy from school checked out that Web site. He saw our pictures and decided to distribute them around school! To make things even worse, the administration found out about it and contacted our parents. I lost my computer privileges for months. My parents only allowed me to do my homework on the computer, and they also had to be present when I did it.

Self-esteem also plays a role in peer pressure. A person's self-esteem helps influence whether that person will give in to peer pressure or resist it. According to the March of Dimes, self-esteem is defined as a "combination of feeling loved and capable." Self-esteem also refers to a person's self-worth or opinion of oneself, and having negative opinions about oneself is an indication of low self-esteem.

SOCIAL NETWORKING AND PEER PRESSURE

Authors of a 2009 article in the *International Journal of Information Management* looked at factors that influence how much information is disclosed on social networking Web sites. They collected information on students between the ages of 12 and 18. Peer pressure played a significant role on how much information was disclosed. The stronger the peer pressure, the more likely adolescents were to disclose personal information. That makes sense because social networks are designed to let friends and family communicate with each other.

Similar results were found by the authors of an article in a 2009 issue of *CyberPsychology and Behavior*. In this study, college students indicated they felt pressured by friends to join Facebook. A 2009 study in *New Media & Society* produced the same results. The authors found that students felt pressured to join Facebook or risk having their social lives suffer. In at least one instance, a friend signed someone else up in order to "encourage" participation.

CYBER-BULLYING AND PEER PRESSURE

Research is missing on the link between peer pressure and other online behaviors. However, some preliminary insights can be made, which surely will be followed up by academic research in the upcoming years.

One of the most obvious connections is between peer pressure and cyber-bullying. There is some evidence that peer pressure influences bullying behavior. Authors of a 2008 study in *Qualitative Health Research* looked at the relationship between peer pressure and bullying and found that students often felt compelled to participate in bullying behavior. Some students indicated they joined in the bullying to maintain a sense of belonging to a social group. At a minimum, many students would not intervene in the incident to avoid the appearance of deviating from the group's norms. Cyber-bullying is often an extension of in-person bullying. Therefore, it makes sense that members of a peer group will continue such behavior in an online setting.

RESISTING PEER PRESSURE

Peer pressure is a fact of life. It is important to know ways to stand up to peer pressure in order to avoid making regrettable mistakes. The most important step is to say no. This means a person needs to let the group know his or her feelings and that engaging in the behavior is not the right thing to do. Walking away from a situation may be called for.

TEENS SPEAK

Turns Out My "Friends" Were Just Users

I learned that my friends weren't really friends. They just liked to use people to get things they wanted. I didn't know any better. They were considered the cool group in school. One day a few of them started talking to me. Over a couple of weeks I ended up hanging out with them. It was great! I felt like I was becoming a part of the cool group. The fun lasted for a while and then they started pressuring me into do things I didn't like. They would have me help them cheat on tests. Then I was asked to help shoplift items—nothing major, but it was still stealing. That's not what my parents taught me. After the second time I did that, I decided it was enough. I told them it wasn't cool and if we got caught we'd be in a lot of trouble. They started questioning my loyalty to the group. That's when it occurred to me that I was just being used. They didn't care what kind of person I was. I either played their game or I wasn't going to be part of their group. That disgusted me, and I ended up walking away. I'm glad I did. About a month later they were busted for stealing clothes from a store. They may be the "cool" kids, but they've got a police record. I don't.

A person who constantly faces pressure to participate in risky or problem behaviors needs to reevaluate her friends. It may be time to look for new friends. Either the person does not have much in common with the group or the person's values and beliefs no longer match that of the group. Although many teenagers do it, it makes no sense to be part of a group that engages in questionable behavior.

Another way to resist peer pressure is to build and maintain a high level of self-esteem. Self-esteem helps people realize they do not always need the approval of others to be happy. This means not worrying about losing some friends because others will come along. High self-esteem also helps people realize they do not have to go along with questionable behavior in order to be liked.

Maintaining a diverse group of friends can help mediate the influences of peer pressure. Some friends may disagree with certain behaviors, while other friends are for those behaviors. Losing some friends because a person does not give in to peer pressure can be less bothersome because there are still other friends around. A person will not be socially isolated. It is also recommended that a person's friends be able to make their own decisions. Being friends with others who can resist peer pressure increases the chances of avoiding peer pressure altogether. Other people who are not interested in being subjected to peer pressure will be less likely to exert that pressure on others.

Of course, resisting peer pressure is easier said than done. It takes work to stand up to others. Someone who does not have high self-esteem will also need to work at that. Also, no one likes to be criticized or bullied. Even though peer pressure will not last forever, it can feel like it will at the time. Ultimately, people must follow their conscience and do the right thing.

See also: Bullies and Cyber-bullying; Prevention; Surfing and Online Communication; Social Networking Web Sites

FURTHER READING

Prinstein, Mitchell J., and Kenneth A. Dodge. *Understanding Peer Influence in Children and Adolescents.* New York: Guilford Press, 2010.
Tarshis, Thomas Paul. *Living With Peer Pressure and Bullying.* New York: Checkmark Books, 2010.

■ PHISHING AND PHARMING

Techniques to defraud victims by illegally obtaining their personal information. This information then can be used to commit identity theft. Phishing involves sending potential victims an e-mail, typically indicating that the person needs to provide personal information for verification of an account. People who follow through unknowingly provide financial information to offenders. Pharming is more dangerous than phishing because e-mail is not used. Attackers target vulnerabilities in Web sites, which results in sending potential victims to a similar-looking Web site. People then enter personal information, thinking they are on the proper Web site. Offenders then use this information to commit identity theft.

PHISHING

The Anti-Phishing Working Group (APWG) defines *phishing* as "a criminal mechanism employing both social engineering and technical subterfuge to steal consumers' personal data and financial account credentials." In other words, phishing is an illegal attempt to collect confidential information from a person in order to access accounts and steal funds.

According to the author of an article in a 2010 issue of the *Journal of Computer Security,* a phishing Web site is online for an average of three days. The author also notes that many Web sites disappear after a few hours.

The author distinguishes between two types of phishing attacks: malware-based phishing and deceptive phishing. Malware-based attacks do not need potential victims to provide information; software is spread by e-mail (the same way computer viruses are spread). The software then tries to install itself on a computer. If successful, it will search the computer for sensitive information and transmit that back to the phisher.

Deceptive phishing is what most people think of when they hear the term "phishing." According to the author there are a number of tactics that can be used to phish for information. These include: **social engineering, mimicry, e-mail spoofing, URL hiding, invisible content,** and image content.

Mimicry is one reason many phishing scams work. E-mails and any related Web sites are designed to look official. For example, a phisher may target people who use a certain credit card or bank. The e-mails are designed to look like they came from the institution. The Web site will be a copy, or a very similar version, of the real company's Web site. All of this is done to minimize the chances that victims will realize they are being targeted.

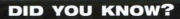

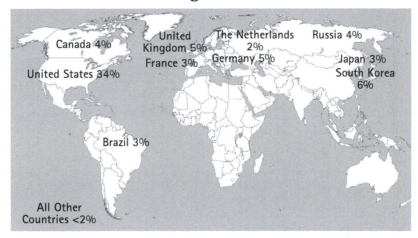

Location of Phishing Scams, 2010

Canada 4%

United Kingdom 5%

The Netherlands 2%

Russia 4%

France 3%

Germany 5%

Japan 3%

United States 34%

South Korea 6%

Brazil 3%

All Other Countries <2%

As of January 2010, the majority of phishing attacks originated in the United States.

Source: PhishTank. http://www.phishtank.com. Accessed February 27, 2010.

E-mail spoofing and URL hiding are similar to mimicry. An e-mail spoof hides the sender's identity by providing a fake sender e-mail address. Similarly, URL hiding involves making links in an e-mail look legitimate, while hiding the real URL address.

Phishing scams take a large financial toll. The author of a 2007 article in *Info Security* conservatively estimates that more than $320 million is lost every year because of phishing scams. In the same year, the Gartner Group estimated that $2 billion was lost because of phishing.

PHARMING

According to the Web site SearchSecurity.com, "Pharming is a scamming practice in which **malicious code** is installed on a personal computer or server, misdirecting users to fraudulent Web sites without their knowledge or consent."

Unlike phishing, where an e-mail is sent to lure a victim to a Web site, pharming attacks legitimate sites to send potential victims to

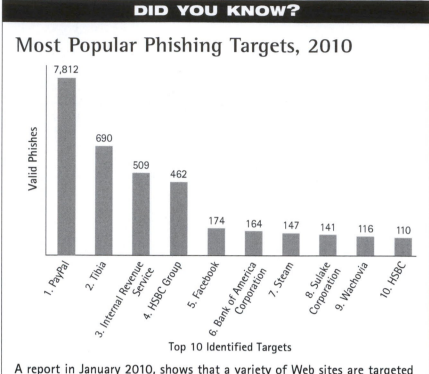

DID YOU KNOW?

Most Popular Phishing Targets, 2010

A report in January 2010, shows that a variety of Web sites are targeted in phishing attacks. Even the Web site for the U.S. Internal Revenue Service is a popular target.

Source: PhishTank. http://www.phishtank.com. Accessed February 27, 2010.

fraudulent sites. For example, a user may go to her regular bank's Web site, such as www.example.bank.com. Because the pharmer has attacked the Web site, it sends people to a different site without the potential victims knowing. This makes it very easy to gather personal information, because the victim still believes he or she is on a legitimate Web site.

Pharming v. phishing

As the authors of a 2009 article in *Applied Intelligence* state, it is harder to detect pharming attacks than phishing attacks. Pharming is considered more dangerous than phishing. The media has provided sufficient coverage of phishing attacks so Internet users may have a better understanding of what constitutes a fraudulent e-mail. Still, there are many victims who fall for phishing scams. Further, there are fewer, if any, warning signs that you are going to be a victim of a pharming scheme. Pharming can be more dangerous because of fewer, if any, warning signs.

Drive-by pharming

There is a form of pharming called **drive-by pharming**, which occurs when a user visits a Web site with malicious code. The programming code is able to change the *user's* Internet settings so when a person visit's a Web site, she or he can be redirected to a pharmer's Web site. This is possible when users do not have proper security settings on their routers. A person who has created a secure, password-protected home network is fine. However, most people do not do this, leaving themselves exposed to potential attacks.

Getting protection

Unfortunately, protection from pharming is difficult to achieve. Companies with Internet Web sites need to use security software to help prevent their sites from pharming attacks. However, users can take some preventative measures against pharming. According to the Web site pharming.org, users should only use pharming-conscious Web sites. These are sites that use security protocols to process transactions. If a user goes to a secure Web site that is being attacked, that person will receive a message from the Internet browser that the security certificate does not match the Internet address the person is using. The browser will ask the user if he wants to proceed using the Web site. It is recommended that the user click the "Never" option to avoid the possibility of being a pharming victim.

See also: Internet Safety; Prevention; Privacy Issues; Surfing and Online Communication

FURTHER READING

James, Lance. *Phishing Exposed.* Burlington, Mass.: Syngress, 2006.
Long, Johnny, and Jack Wiles. *No Tech Hacking.* Burlington, Mass.: Syngress, 2008.
Viega, John. *The Myths of Security: What the Computer Security Industry Doesn't Want You to Know.* Sebastopol, Calif.: O'Reilly, 2009.

■ PHYSICAL THREATS

The promise of physical violence sent over the Internet. E-mail, instant messages, chat rooms, and forums allow people to threaten each other. Physical threats are meant to scare and control the recipient because of the threat of bodily harm.

ONLINE THREATS

Unfortunately, there is not yet any good research on the topic of physical threats that occur over the Internet. Even the research on bullying typically does not distinguish between physical and other types of threats. Obviously such threats do occur. However, the frequency of these threats is unknown, as is hard data on offenders and victims.

An e-mail scam known as the Hitman Scam has grown in popularity. The Internet Crime Complaint Center received numerous complaints about this type of scam, in which potential victims receive an e-mail from a hitman. The e-mail indicates this person has been hired to assassinate the victim. However, the hitman is willing to buy the person's safety if the potential victim sends money. The money needs to be sent to the hitman within two to three days; otherwise the assassination attempt will take place. This type of scam capitalizes on the phrase your money or your life.

Authors of a 2007 article in the *Journal of Adolescent Health* provide some insight into the frequency of physical threats over the Internet. The authors found that 4 percent of teenagers who were 16 or 17 years old had been harassed in a manner that was distressing. This meant that the teenagers had either been threatened online or harassed in a way that caused them to be extremely upset. One problem, however, is the authors did not distinguish between threats and harassment. Further, a threat received online may or may not have a physical component. For example, a person could threaten to share sensitive information with other people. Or someone might threaten to beat up the student at school the next day. Both are threats; however, the nature of the threats differ. One is physical while the other is psychological, intending to have a negative impact on one's emotional well-being.

DEALING WITH THREATS

There are several things people can do to help prevent and deal with threats. First, it is important to know who is making the threats. If the threat comes from someone the user knows, it should be taken more seriously. When threats come from people at school, work, or the local area, it is easier to carry them out. Conversely, threats that come from people who live hundreds or thousands of miles away are much less likely to actually occur.

Anytime a threat is made, a person should print it out. In this way there is documentation of the threat. Threats should be reported to authorities. If the user making the threats is unknown to the victim, then it may be difficult for the police to do anything. However, if the offender is known to the victim then the police know whom to deal with. Further, if there is a positive identification of the offender and proof that threats were made, the offender's Internet service provider can disable the Internet connection. People who have been caught downloading pirated music can be disconnected by their Internet providers for violating the company's terms of use.

It is not wise to threaten the person who made the original threats. That can escalate the problem, and the victim also can get into trouble. It is much better to stop talking with the person. Unlike the physical world where it may be difficult to walk away from a threat, all someone has to do over the Internet is block the offender, switch to a different Web site, or shut off the computer.

See also: Bullies and Cyber-bullying; Hate Crimes and Online Predators; Internet Safety; Surfing and Online Communication

FURTHER READING

McQuade III, Samuel C., James P. Colt, and Nancy Meyer. *Cyber Bullying: Protecting Kids and Adults From Online Bullies.* Santa Barbara, Calif.: Praeger, 2009.

Roddel, Victoria. *The Ultimate Guide to Internet Safety.* Raleigh, N.C.: Lulu.com, 2009.

Trolley, Barbara C., and Constance Hanel. *Cyber Kids, Cyber Bullying, Cyber Balance.* Thousand Oaks, Calif.: Corwin, 2009.

■ PORNOGRAPHY AND ONLINE PREDATORS

Creative activity of no artistic value other than to stimulate sexual desire and its influence on online predators. Pornography is a large business, drawing in more than $2 billion in Internet sales alone. Further, there are thousands of Web sites with free pornography.

This includes child pornography. Research has shown relationships do exist between the use of pornography and sexual aggression, but there is no hard research yet on the relationship between the use of pornography and online predatory behaviors. Research on Internet offenders has focused instead on the possession, distribution, and creation of pornography and child pornography.

THE PORNOGRAPHY INDUSTRY

There is an immeasurable amount of pornography on the Internet. The industry is gigantic. As of 2010, the latest available statistics indicate that there is more than $13 billion in revenue, according to a 2009 report by CNBC on the pornography industry. The report also indicates that approximately $2.84 billion of the revenue comes from Internet sales.

A 2006 report, from the *Internet Filter Review,* indicates that revenue from pornography across the world is an estimated $97 billion per year. The CNBC report also indicates that the industry is starting to lose revenue because of the Internet. Piracy of videos is rampant, and there are thousands of Web sites that let people view porn for free or a fee.

PORNOGRAPHY AND SEXUAL OFFENDING

A very limited amount of research shows that some offenders use pornography during a crime. Unfortunately the evidence is not recent. Authors of a 2004 article in the *International Journal of Offender Therapy and Comparative Criminology* examined this question. Forty-seven percent of offenders had pornography in their possession during a crime. However, the authors found that only 17 percent of offenders in their sample used pornography as part of the crime.

Looking at only those offenders who used pornography during a crime, 55 percent had shown the material to the victim. Another 37 percent had taken pictures of the victim during the crime, which constitutes the creation of pornography. Finally, the remaining 13 percent had used pornography right before the crime to become stimulated.

Some other results are worth noting. Almost 26 percent of offenders who victimized children outside the family had used pornography. This compares to almost 17 percent of offenders who committed incest.

A 2008 study in *Aggressive Behavior* indicates that pornography may not be as influential as people suspect when it comes to aggressive behavior in general. The authors review evidence that certain types of pornography have different affects on sexual offending. For example, seeing nudity actually decreased aggression. However, both nonviolent and violent sexual behavior increased aggression.

When analyzing their own data, the authors found that pornography is not as strongly linked to sexual aggression as some people's behavior. The authors did find a relationship between pornography and sexual aggression. That relationship was significantly weakened once a person's propensity for sexual aggression was taken into account. In other words, once the likelihood of a person being sexually aggressive was looked at, pornography became less of a factor.

A 2009 study in *BMC Psychiatry* presented information on the relationship between viewing Internet child pornography and sexual offending. The authors found that only 3.5 percent of child pornography "consumers" had convictions for nonviolent sexual offenses, such as being in the possession of illegal pornography. Only one percent had been previously convicted of child sexual abuse.

The authors of a article in a 2009 issues of the *Journal of Family Violence* found that it was common for Internet sexual offenders to have sexually assaulted children. In their study of convicted offenders, 74 percent had no documented cases of sexually abusing a child. However, by the end of a treatment program for sex offenders, 85 percent of offenders indicated they had sexually abused a child. Further, of the remaining 15 percent, which was 24 offenders, only two offenders passed a polygraph that indicated they had not abused a child in the past. Out of 155 offenders in the program, there were only two offenders who had not been involved in prior abuse.

PORNOGRAPHY AND ONLINE CRIMES

Although it has been shown that viewing pornography is related to sexual aggression, the question remains whether pornography influences the behavior of online predators. That question is much more difficult to answer because there is limited research on the subject. Research has focused on offenders who possess child pornography.

CHILD PORNOGRAPHY

Child pornography is estimated to be a multibillion dollar business. The author of an article in a 2009 issue of the *Scientific World*

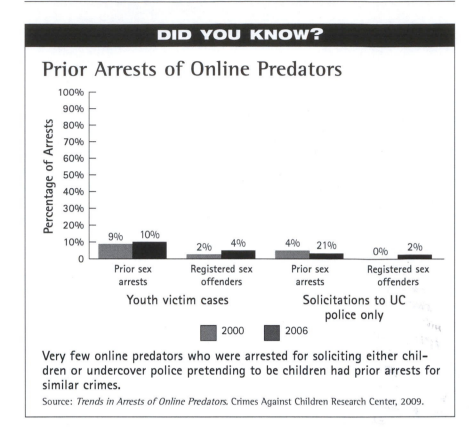

DID YOU KNOW?

Prior Arrests of Online Predators

Very few online predators who were arrested for soliciting either children or undercover police pretending to be children had prior arrests for similar crimes.

Source: *Trends in Arrests of Online Predators.* Crimes Against Children Research Center, 2009.

Journal found that there are several thousand Internet Web sites dedicated to child pornography. At the time of the author's review, he indicated that 54 percent of these Web sites were located in the United States. Given the frequency with which Web sites are taken down and put up, however, it is difficult to estimate how accurate that figure is today.

Authors of a 2007 in the *Journal of Adolescent Health* examined how often youth received requests for sexual pictures. The authors found that 4 percent of children between the ages of 10 and 17 had received online requests for these pictures. Luckily, only one person actually followed through with the request. Girls were almost four times more likely than boys to receive these requests. Children who were black were three times more likely than white children to receive requests.

TEENS SPEAK

It Was Fun at First . . .

It's fun to be flirty on the Internet. I mean, how many people are really going to take it seriously? I would talk with people in chat rooms and using Yahoo! Instant Messenger. There would be times I would get chat requests from guys looking for cybersex. In many cases I decided to play along. After all, these people tend to be pathetic. Why not make fun of them?

I ended up stopping these actions. In one case I was sent pictures of a guy posing naked. It was gross. Seriously, why would anyone want to do that? It's embarrassing. This guy wasn't a model or that good looking. Then, to make things worse, he started asking me for nude pictures. When I refused to play along, he became nasty, calling me a tease and cyber-slut. The comments kept coming and I ended up having to block him from contacting me through instant messenger. Luckily he didn't have my e-mail address so I didn't have to worry about getting mean e-mails. After that experience, I decided it wasn't worth playing around with people I don't know.

Children talking with people they met online and had not met in person were more than five times more likely to receive requests for sexual pictures. Adults were almost four times more likely to ask other children to request sexual pictures. However, the most telling statistic indicates that adults who sent the children a sexual picture were nearly 10 times more likely to ask for a picture in return.

Traits of child pornographers

In a 2007 issue of *Sex Abuse,* the authors of an article examined the characteristics of offenders convicted of possessing Internet child pornography. The authors found that 92 percent of the offenders had no prior sexual offense convictions. Four percent had a prior conviction for a sexual offense involving a child, while one person involved an adult victim. The remaining offenders had been convicted of a crime that did not involve being in physical contact with a victim (for example, possession of illegal pornography). The authors also indicate that Internet offenders are less likely to have prior sexual convictions when compared to child molesters. In this case, 20 percent of child molesters had prior sexual offense convictions involving a child.

The authors did find that Internet offenders had between two and 921,000 images in their possession at the time of arrest. This averages out to 16,698 images per offender. However, that number is inflated because some offenders had several hundred thousand images in their possession. Another measure found that offenders had approximately 317 images in their possession.

SOME CONCLUSIONS

Our understanding about sexual offenders on the Internet is limited. Over the past decade, there have not been many studies on the subject. Most of the studies that have been published focus on offenders arrested for the possession, creation, and distribution of child pornography through the Internet.

Studies that look at the relationship between pornography and online predatory behavior do not exist. Although there is a relationship between pornography and sexual aggression, this relationship cannot be extended to online behaviors of sexual predators. To better understand how pornography may influence online predatory behaviors, new research is needed.

See also: Internet Safety; Online Predators, Characteristics of; Online Victimization, Examples of; Sexual Predators, Online

FURTHER READING

Arnaldo, Carlos A. *Child Abuse on the Internet: Ending the Silence.* New York: Berghahn Books, 2001.

Attwood, Feona. *Porn.com: Making Sense of Online Pornography.* New York: Peter Lang Publishing Group, 2009.

Sandler, Corey. *Living With the Internet and Online Dangers.* New York: Facts On File, 2010.

■ PREJUDICE AND ONLINE BEHAVIOR

Influence on online behavior of a preconceived idea, belief, or attitude that can lead to abusive acts. Because the Internet facilitates communication around the world, it is easy to share prejudices about various groups. Although little research thus far has been devoted to this subject, some evidence indicates that prejudicial or biased comments are common in the online world. Prejudicial remarks such as hate speech are protected by the First Amendment of the Constitution.

PREJUDICE ON THE INTERNET

Anonymity allows people to explore and voice their prejudices. Because views can be expressed without being linked to a specific individual, the potential for consequences or punishments is greatly reduced. Because the Internet is a communications medium, prejudices that occur in the physical world can be brought into the virtual world.

Social networking Web sites are designed to allow people to connect with each other. Social networks can be based on prejudicial attitudes. As of 2010, for example, it is possible to find groups on Facebook dedicated to white supremacy. In fact, Web sites based on prejudice and hate abound on the Internet. Hate groups even have their own Web sites, which allow them to spread their messages.

Racial discrimination

Authors of a 2008 study in the *Journal of Adolescent Health* found that racial discrimination was a common experience among students. The authors found that 71 percent of African Americans and 71 percent of whites found examples of racial discrimination online that were degrading to their race or ethnicity. There was no direct attack against the user.

The authors also found that 29 percent of African Americans were individually discriminated against online. This involved saying something against the user because she or he belonged to a specific racial or ethnic group. Twenty percent of whites experienced individual discrimination, while 42 percent of multiracial youth had this type of experience. It was found that 50 percent of these experiences occurred on social networking Web sites. Text messages, instant messages, chat rooms, and discussion forums were also online locations where discrimination occurred.

An older study, published in a 2004 issue of *Applied Developmental Psychology,* provides some insight into prejudice and online behavior. The authors of this study examined comments made in teen chat rooms. The authors studied comments made in monitored and unmonitored chat rooms. They found that in monitored chat rooms, negative comments about racial or ethnic groups made up 19 percent of all comments. In *un*monitored chat rooms, 59 percent of comments were negative and directed toward racial or ethnic groups.

There are no recent studies that examine if prejudicial attitudes influence online behavior. This is one of many areas that needs to be studied. Generally, prejudice can influence online behavior in one of two ways. First, users can avoid biased Web sites and chat rooms as well as discussions with people who make prejudicial responses. If a user does not like the content, it is easy to simply avoid the Web site. Users who advocate tolerance can avoid Web sites that demean groups or promote hate. At the same time, a person with certain prejudices can avoid Web sites that go against their views.

Second, sadly, users can seek opportunities to share their prejudices with others by making derogatory remarks in forums or chat rooms or finding people to harass through instant messaging or e-mail. Whatever the method, the Internet allows people to express their prejudices and lash out at members of target groups. Because hate speech is protected by the U.S. Constitution, even prejudiced individuals can promote their views without fear of censorship or legal consequences.

See also: Hate Crimes and Online Predators; Surfing and Online Communication

FURTHER READING
Chakraborti, Neil. *Hate Crime: Concepts, Policy, Future Directions.* Devon, U.K.: Willan Publishing, 2010.
Cimino, Michelle. *NETiquette (On-line Etiquette): Tips for Adults & Teens: Facebook, MySpace, Twitter! Terminology . . . and More.* Frederick, Md.: PublishAmerica, 2009.

■ PREVALENCE AND STATISTICS

Recorded frequency of events or behavior. Over the past decade, Internet use has significantly grown. Teenagers spend close to 27 hours per week on the Internet.

Opportunities for social networking have grown, with social network Web sites being among the most popular sites online. Facebook has more than 100 million unique visitors per month. As the online world has grown, so have opportunities to victimize people. Child pornography has flourished, with an estimated 100,000 Web sites available to find material. Bullying has also migrated to the Internet, with approximately 11 percent of students being victimized. Identity thieves also use the Internet to find victims. E-mail is the most common method to make contact with potential victims.

INTERNET USE

The Web site Internet World Stats provides data on Internet use around the world. According to data from the Web site, 25.6 percent of the world's population uses the Internet. This may seem low until you remember that people in many countries, especially many third world countries, have little or no Internet access. For example, only 6.8 percent of the African population has Internet access. In Asia, only 19.4 percent of the population has access. By comparison, 74.2 percent of the North American population accesses the Internet.

Education and use

A 2010 report by the Pew Research Center provides similar results. According to the study, 74 percent of American adults use the Internet. For both men and women, 74 percent use the Internet. Education also plays a role in Internet use. Ninety-four percent of college graduates use the Internet, compared to only 39 percent of people who did not graduate from high school.

Age and use

A 2010 report by the Kaiser Family Foundation examined media use among kids and teenagers between the ages of eight and 18. In 1999, only 47 percent of this group had access to the Internet from home. By 2009, that number had increased to 84 percent. Access from a teen's bedroom increased from 10 percent in 1999 to 33 percent by 2009. A 2009 report by Cox Communications found that teenagers between the ages of 13 and 18 spent an average of 26.8 hours *per week* using the Internet. Also included in this average was time spent online for schoolwork.

SOCIAL NETWORKING DATA

Social networks are an extremely popular form of communicating with friends, as well as a way of making new friends. Web sites such as Facebook, MySpace, Friendster, Twitter, and numerous online dating sites collectively attract hundreds of millions of visitors each month.

ComScore, a company that tracks online behavior, indicated that in December 2009 there were approximately 112 million unique visitors to Facebook. Compete.com, another company that tracks Internet statistics, indicated that in January 2010 there were more than 133 million visitors to Facebook. Although it is difficult to obtain a precise measure of visitors to Web sites such as Facebook, because different companies collect data differently, an August 17, 2009, blog post found on Econsultancy.com put Facebook's popularity into perspective: "If Facebook were a country, it would be the fourth most populated place in the world."

Other social networking sites have proven to be popular. However, Facebook has overtaken them all. For example, comScore estimates that in January 2010 there were 70 million MySpace users located in the United States. Compete.com estimates that there were slightly more than 49 million unique visitors to MySpace in December 2009. As of January 2010, Myspace was the second most popular social networking Web site, while Twitter came in at number three. Twitter attracted approximately 22.8 million unique visitors during December 2009.

Although social networking is popular, blogging does not appear to be very popular among teenagers. A 2010 report by the Pew Internet & American Life Project found that only 14 percent of online teens blogged during 2009. This is a 50 percent drop from 2006, when 28 percent of online teens were blogging. Similar results were found in a 2009 study by Cox Communications. The company found that only 12 percent of teenagers between the ages of 13 and 18 had blogged in the prior 30 days.

ONLINE DATA FOR PREDATORS

It is not possible to determine the prevalence of online predators in the general public. However, there is some data on predators who have been arrested. Online predators are male and tend to be at least 35 years old. Authors of a 2007 article in *Psychology, Crime & Law* found that 73 percent of the offenders in their study were employed. Almost 47 percent were either married or in a relationship.

Child pornographers are a common type of Internet predator. In a 2009 article found in *TheScientificWorldJournal*, the author indicated there are several thousand Web sites dedicated to child pornography. Some estimate that more than 100,000 such Web sites exist. The authors of an article in a 2007 issue of the *Journal of Adolescent Health* found that 4 percent of children between the ages of 10 and 17 had been solicited online for sexual pictures. Girls were four times more likely to receive these requests. In a 2007 article found in *Psychology, Crime & Law,* the authors learned that 83 percent of convicted Internet sex offenders had primarily viewed female child pornography. The author of a 2007 study in the *Journal of Child Sexual Abuse* found that 52 percent of Internet sex offenders would send child pornography to children with whom they chatted online.

A 2009 report by the Crimes Against Children Research Center is one of the few reports that has examined changes over time in arrests of online predators. In 2000, 664 arrests were made by police officers who had pretended to be children online. When offenders went to meet these kids, the police arrested them. In 2006, there were 3,100 such arrests, a 381 percent increase.

DATA ON CYBER-BULLYING

Cyber-bullying is abusive behavior conducted through the Internet or cell phones. It can consist of threats, demeaning messages, publicly posting embarrassing comments or pictures, sharing private information, and so forth. Computers even can be damaged if bullies successfully infect them with a virus.

Authors of a 2008 article in the *Scandinavian Journal of Psychology* found that 11.7 of students had been victims of cyber-bullying. Slightly more than 17 percent of students between 12 and 15 had been victims, while 3.3 percent of students between 15 and 20 were victims.

A 2009 article in *New Media & Society* reported similar findings. The authors reported that 11.1 percent of students had been victims. In this study the most common forms of cyber-bullying were making threats and insults.

Cyber-bullying does not appear to be a random act. In a 2009 article found in *School Psychology International,* the authors reported that the most common reason for cyber-bullying was a dislike of the person. Authors of a 2009 study in the *Journal of Educational Administration* found that 91 percent of incidents were a result of relationship problems.

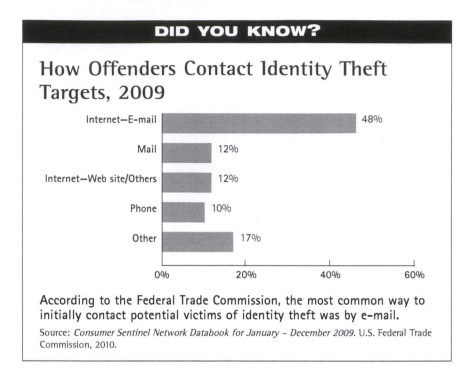

DID YOU KNOW?

How Offenders Contact Identity Theft Targets, 2009

According to the Federal Trade Commission, the most common way to initially contact potential victims of identity theft was by e-mail.

Source: *Consumer Sentinel Network Databook for January – December 2009*. U.S. Federal Trade Commission, 2010.

IDENTITY THEFT

The Internet provides many opportunities for identity theft to occur. Offenders use fraudulent techniques to obtain personal information from victims, such as social security numbers or account numbers. It is hard to determine the extent of the financial consequences associated with online identity theft.

A 2010 report by the Federal Trade Commission indicates that credit card fraud is the most common form of reported identity theft. This accounts for 17 percent of reported identity thefts. Bank fraud accounted for 10 percent of complaints and loan fraud constituted another 4 percent. Government documents/benefits fraud accounted for 16 percent of complaints, while employment fraud accounted for 13 percent of complaints. Finally, phone or utilities fraud made up 15 percent of complaints.

See also: Blogging; Bullies and Cyber-bullying; Online Predators, Characteristics of; Phishing and Pharming; Sexual Predators, Online; Social Networking Web Sites

FURTHER READING
Christakis, Nicholas A., and James H. Fowler. *Connected: The Surprising Power of Our Social Networks and How They Shape Our Lives.* New York: Little, Brown and Company, 2009.
Salter, Anna. *Predators: Pedophiles, Rapists, and Other Sex Offenders.* Jackson, Tenn.: Basic Books, 2004.
Sullivan, Mike. *Online Predators.* Longwood, Fla.: Xulon Press, 2008.

■ PREVENTION

Measures to deter online harassment. Internet users can take steps to help prevent online problems. Antivirus software can help prevent malware from being installed on a personal computer. Limiting personal information can make it difficult for others to determine a user's identity and location. Internet etiquette also can help prevent others from getting angry and attempting to retaliate.

PREVENTIVE MEASURES

There are several steps a user can take to prevent computer attacks, harassment, and sexual solicitation. One of the best ways to prevent a computer from being infected with malware is to install antivirus and anti-spyware software. Some software companies sell "security suite" programs that contain everything needed to protect a computer from outside intrusion. This software can make it extremely difficult for personal information to be stolen off a home computer via the Internet. In turn this reduces the risk of identity theft.

Personal information

Another measure that can be used to help prevent problems is to limit the amount of personal information that is shared online. Social networking Web sites have exploded in popularity, with Facebook being the most popular. These Web sites allow users to share information with others. This information can be restricted to certain friends or it can be shared with anyone who looks at a user's profile. Social networking sites allow people to connect with other people who have similar friends and interests. In order to meet other people, a person will have to divulge a little information, such as interests or careers. Sharing too much personal information immediately creates an opportunity for abuse by others. Giving strangers access to a home address or telephone number can potentially lead to harassment or stalking.

Another way to help prevent problems online is to use benign screen names when in chat rooms or on an instant messenger program. Provocative names that include swear words or sexual references attract attention. This includes attracting the attention of online sexual predators. The author of a 2007 study in the *Journal of Child Sexual Abuse* studied how sex offenders identified and contacted minors over the Internet. Offenders would look at screen names and the comments of users. If either made any reference to sex, that would catch the attention of offenders. If a screen name possibly indicated the user was young, that also would catch a predator's attention.

Online interactions and netiquette

Another way to help prevent problems online is to use Internet etiquette, referred to as **netiquette.** When using instant messaging, chat rooms, or e-mail, be civil to others. This means be careful not to abuse your "power." In a recent interview, Kathleen Taylor, author of *Cruelty: Human Evil and the Human Brain,* explained: "We developed to have constant [face-to-face] feedback from others, telling us if it was O.K. to be saying what we're saying. On the Internet, you get nothing, no body language, no gesture. So you get this feeling of unlimited power because there is nothing stopping you, no instant feedback."

Avoid derogatory remarks, and do not engage in **flaming.** If others engage in this behavior, they can be blocked. Instant messaging programs allow people to block specific users. Many online chat rooms also have this feature and use the delete key if nasty e-mails arrive.

See also: Chat Rooms and Instant Messaging; Internet Safety; Online Victimization, Examples of; Phishing and Pharming; Privacy Issues; Social Networking Web Sites

FURTHER READING
Kelsey, Todd. *Social Networking Spaces.* New York: Apress, 2010.
Roddel, Victoria. *The Ultimate Guide to Internet Safety.* Raleigh, N.C.: Lulu.com, 2009.

■ PRIVACY ISSUES

Protection of personal information on the Internet. With the increasing role the Internet plays in peoples' lives, everyone is concerned about privacy. How much information should a person share? How much information is a company allowed to gather? Should companies be able to track users' Web activity to gather information for marketing purposes?

How much of a right to privacy should people expect when they use the Internet? Web sites such as Facebook and Google have been severely scrutinized for their privacy policies. Using Web sites that provide services such as online storage and word processing also have privacy implications.

FACEBOOK AND PRIVACY

Facebook has been subjected to lawsuits over privacy issues. Facebook made changes to their privacy options toward the end of 2009, so that users would gain more control over what others could see.

Further, users claimed that the new "recommended" settings allowed too much private information to be shared. In order to fix this, a user would have to adjust the settings. Accepting the recommended settings would make public a user's photos and wall posts. The author of an article on CNET, published on December 9, 2009, indicated that a user's political and religious views would be shared with that user's extended network (friends of friends).

According to the Electronic Frontier Foundation, Facebook's updated privacy policies were intended to make users share more information. The EFF also states that the recommended privacy settings display more information unless a user goes through and changes each setting.

The EFF and others suggested more restrictive default settings. This would prevent users from accidentally allowing the public to see information that should have remained private. It would then be the user's responsibility to alter the settings so more people could see select information.

Who takes responsibility?

This raises the question as to who is responsible for the privacy settings. Is it Facebook's responsibility to protect people from accidentally sharing information? Or is it each user's responsibility to make sure all privacy settings are accurate? Ultimately, each user is responsible for content posted and who can see that content. Arguments that Facebook is trying to push people to share more content are accurate. However, Facebook is a company, and companies need to find ways to continue making money; sharing content is one way to attract new users.

When do people share information?

Two researchers from Cambridge University in England presented a paper on privacy issues with social networks in 2009 at the Eighth Workshop on the Economics of Information Security. One aspect of the authors' work focused on a concept known as **privacy salience,** or **privacy-priming.** Privacy salience refers to the negative effect privacy policies can have on information sharing. The authors found that people are less likely to share information when they know strong privacy policies are in place. It does not sound right: People should be *more* willing to share information when they are assured that information will be protected. However, think about the type of information that is shared when registering with a social networking Web site. The information provided does not seem to be that sensitive. If that is what people believe, then they question why a company would need such a strong privacy policy. After all, if "there's nothing to worry about," then why would a strong policy be needed? This makes users suspicious and more protective.

As a result, companies actually can hurt their goals by being upfront about their privacy policies. People may not be as willing to sign up, or if they do, then they may not be as forthcoming about personal information. For social networking sites, that can hurt business.

The authors also discuss **privacy negotiations.** This refers to the tradeoff a person must make when using a social networking Web site. A person can use the site for free; in return, a person has to provide information that can be used for a variety of purposes. The question one needs to ask is, "Is this site worth giving private information to the company that runs it?"

The author of a special report found on Economist.com summarizes this issue best when stating "How much is a free lunch?"

The author also makes the following observation: Web sites promote content-sharing and downplay privacy policies. The reason is simple—it is difficult to move content from one Web site to another.

DID YOU KNOW?

Complaints to the Federal Trade Commission

The Federal Trade Commission received approximately five times as many complaints in 2008 as they did in 2000. In 2008, almost 319,000 calls were complaints about identity theft.

Source: Consumer Sentinel Network Databook for January 2008-December 2008. U.S. Federal Trade Commission, 2009.

The more content a user produces, the less likely that user will be to leave the Web site for another.

GOOGLE AND PRIVACY

Google has been the subject of numerous privacy complaints. Privacy concerns have surfaced regarding Gmail, Street View, use of cookies, and Google Buzz. For example, Google Buzz is the company's version of social networking. However, Google caused an uproar when the service was launched. The service is linked to Gmail and was initially set up so people could follow everyone in their Gmail contact list.

The problem was the privacy settings were confusing. The service had automatically set up the service for people to follow their contact list. This upset a lot of people because they wanted to pick and choose whom they followed. Although they could change the privacy settings, people wanted the option presented before they started using the service, instead of having to deal with the settings after the fact. In February 2010, Google started correcting the problem.

COMPUTER CLOUDS

One growing aspect of the Internet is the use of computer clouds, an umbrella term used to describe software one uses over the Internet. Web sites such as Google offer services allowing the user to use word processors, spread sheets, e-mail, file storage, and so on. In a sense, all one needs is an Internet connection to do all different kinds of w⁻ If you use a computer cloud service, you can avoid buying   rd for word processors, spreadsheets, PowerPoint, e-mail, and more.

Computer cloud services can be a great convenience. People can work anywhere there is an Internet connection. Cloud computing has proven to be popular. A 2008 report from the Pew Internet & American Life Project indicated that 69 percent of people are using cloud computing services.

Although such computing is convenient, several privacy concerns have been raised. For example, the World Privacy Forum published a report in 2009 that discussed the privacy issues of cloud computing. First, people should be concerned about the security measures these services use to protect data. Users of these services cannot control the company's security features. Although a user assumes the service is secure, one cannot know.

Another issue is the terms of service associated with using cloud computing. People do not usually read these terms. A company may say that to use their cloud computing services, a user gives up certain personal information. This may include information found in the documents stored on the company's server.

Companies offering these services also can be forced to disclose information to the government or private parties. The U.S. Supreme Court says that documents held by a third party, such as a cloud computer service, can be turned over to the government *without* violating a person's right to privacy.

MALWARE

Spyware, a form of malware, has become a problem as well. Malware is defined as a piece of computer code designed to gain access to a computer without the user's permission. According to Symantec, a company that develops security software, spyware can be downloaded from e-mail messages, instant messages, Web sites, and direct file-sharing connections. The company also says that spyware can end up on a person's computer if the person accepts the End User License Agreement when installing a new piece of software. In fact, there has been an increase of malware being transferred by instant messaging. This has led some people to coin the phrase SPIM which is spam for instant messaging.

Ironically, programs designed to prevent and delete spyware from a person's computer may actually be spyware programs. Users should install antivirus and spyware protection software from reputable companies such as AVG, Panda, Symantec, and McAfee, among others.

PERSONAL PRIVACY

Privacy issues go beyond what companies can and cannot do. They also involve friendships over the Internet. What can users expect from other people when they share personal information? Unfortunately, the answer is not much. People can share personal information with the public if they choose.

The author of an article in a January 7, 2010, issue of the *New York Times* discusses the complexities associated with online relationships. The author discusses people's sharing passwords to accounts, such as banking, e-mail, and photo-sharing sites. This sharing is done to help foster intimacy. After all, if users are sharing such personal information, then the other people must be a meaningful part of their lives.

TEENS SPEAK

My Trust Was Completely Violated

I guess I learned the hard way what to share over the Internet. I was dating one guy at school and we e-mailed each other all the time. He'd tell me personal things and I'd share my own thoughts. That included how I felt about other people at school. I really shouldn't have done that. We ended up breaking up, and he got really mad about the whole thing. Then, before I knew it he started sharing my e-mails with people at school. He sent e-mails to people, posted comments on his Facebook page, and even printed e-mails off and gave them to people at school. He made my life really miserable because everyone got mad at me about the things I said. And I couldn't deny them—they were in writing. I lost several friends over that whole ordeal. The next time I date someone I'm not going to share a lot of my personal thoughts through e-mail. I'll either keep them to myself or share them in person. Then, if we break up, I won't have to go through this whole ordeal again.

In 2010, authorities in a school district in Philadelphia, Pennsylvania, got into trouble over privacy issues. The school district had laptop computers for students to use. The students were never told, however, that Webcams could be activated remotely to track the location of laptops in case they went missing. Over a 14-month period, the district activated Webcams 42 times to locate computers. Students sued the school district, claiming the cameras were activated to spy on them. The Federal Bureau of Investigation became involved in the case to see if the district violated computer-intrusion or federal wiretap laws.

See also: Bullies and Cyber-bullying; Peers and Peer Pressure; Social Networking Web Sites

FURTHER READING

Gurak, Laura J. *Persuasion and Privacy in Cyberspace: The Online Protests Over Lotus MarketPlace and the Clipper Chip.* New Haven, Conn.: Yale University Press, 2009.

Jukubiak, David J. *A Smart Kid's Guide to Internet Privacy.* New York: PowerKids Press, 2009.

Rule, James B. *Privacy in Peril: How We Are Sacrificing a Fundamental Right in Exchange for Security and Convenience.* New York: Oxford University Press, 2009.

Solove, Daniel. *The Digital Person: Technology and Privacy in the Information Age.* New York: New York University Press, 2006.

■ SCREEN NAMES

Online identities. Chat rooms, instant messengers, and social networking Web sites, among others, usually require a person to have a screen name. Benign, neutral-sounding screen names are the safest. Screen names with sexual overtones or age references attract online predators.

DEVELOPING A SCREEN NAME

Coming up with a screen name is pretty straightforward. Using a combination of letters, numbers, and symbols, a person creates a unique name. If the name is already taken by another user, a variation of the name, or different name altogether, will be needed.

Using a real name

Many users try to use their own name as a screen name. Unless the screen name is for a social networking Web site, where the person controls the amount of information others can see, it is not recommended that a person use his or her real name. Using a first name may be permissible if it is a common name, such as Chris, Brian, or Meghan. Including a last name in a screen name is too revealing.

Q & A

Question: Can screen names really identify a person?

Answer: Definitely. A *New York Times* article that appeared on March 17, 2010, reported that a person's identity and personal information, such as a birthdate or location, can be identified by finding bits and pieces of information. A screen name itself may not identify a person, unless a real name is used. However, a screen name along with information taken from chat room or instant messenger comments can help a predator to identify a person. That information may lead a predator to search the Internet to find other information and finally piece together a person's identity.

Sexual or age references

Screen names with sexual or age references also lend themselves to abuse. The author of a 2007 study in the *Journal of Child Sexual Abuse* examined how sex offenders identified and contacted minors over the Internet. Offenders would look at screen names and the comments of users. If either made any reference to sex, that would catch the attention of offenders. This is viewed as an indication the user is open to sexual conversation or actions. Predators often will use these types of screen names to let others know they are interested in sexual conversations. If a screen name possibly indicates the user is young, that would also catch a predator's attention. The name tells the predator the user may be naive and open to sexual conversations.

Multiple screen names

Users who visit different chat rooms may want to consider using a different name for each room. People who use the same screen name across various chat rooms, instant messaging programs, and social networking sites may accidentally give too much information to others. In other words, if other users visit the same chat rooms, they may be able to learn more about a person because the screen name is the same. By using different screen names, a greater degree of anonymity is maintained.

Many child pornographers will use this tactic. In order to reduce the likelihood of being arrested, they develop different identities on child pornography Web sites and chat rooms. These offenders are afraid that if one person is arrested, he will be able to identify other child pornographers. To reduce the chances of that happening, offenders change screen names across different Web sites.

Screen names with pictures

Some chat rooms allow people to include a picture next to their screen names. Although the picture is not technically part of the screen name, it obviously provides identifying information to other users. It is not a good idea to include pictures. Predators will then get a better idea about the age and gender of users. Also, avoid provocative pictures, which can have the same effect as screen names with sexual references.

Online identity

Users often feel that screen names are part of their identity. Depending on how deep a person's online life is, this is true. Unfortunately, using such personalized screen names can sometimes be a mistake because of the attention they attract.

Ultimately, users have to be careful with their online conversations, regardless of the screen name. Avoid sharing personal information unless talking with a trusted friend. If a stranger sends a pornographic picture or asks for one, the person is most likely an online predator and should be reported to a responsible adult or authorities.

See also: Blogging; Chat Rooms and Instant Messaging; Internet Safety; Online Predators, Characteristics of; Privacy Issues; Surfing and Online Communication; Sexual Predators, Online; Social Networking Web Sites

FURTHER READING

Bell, Ann. *Exploring Web 2.0: Second Generation Interactive Tools— Blogs, Podcasts, Wikis, Networking, Virtual Worlds, and More.* Scotts Valley, Calif.: CreateSpace, 2009.

Stern, Shayla Thiel. *Instant Identity: Adolescent Girls and the World of Instant Messaging.* New York: Peter Lang Publishing, 2007.

Sullivan, Mike. *Online Predators.* Longwood, Fla.: Xulon Press, 2008.

■ SEXUAL PREDATORS, ONLINE

Someone trying to find a sex partner online in a predatory or abusive manner. There is widespread fear that sexual offenders use the Internet to find victims.

Although there have been numerous high-profile cases where offenders tried or managed to seduce children over the Internet, there is very little research on this group of offenders. Most offenders studied have been arrested for possession of child pornography as child pornography is a widespread problem. Offenders actually engage in countersurveillance techniques to help prevent being arrested. Offenders who do actively search for children focus on usernames to help identify targets. Names that indicate age or reference sex attract the attention of sexual predators.

SEX OFFENDERS

It is extremely difficult to learn about online sex offenders. Aside from sting operations that lure offenders, there are few ways to learn about online behaviors aside from communicating with minors.

Internet versus contact offenders

Authors of a 2009 article in *Sexual Abuse: A Journal of Research and Treatment* examined the psychological profiles of Internet sex offenders and contact sex offenders. Contact sex offenders are those offenders who had direct physical contact with their victims. Internet sex offenders are those who have been convicted of accessing, downloading, trading, or making child pornography. The authors found several differences between contact and Internet offenders. Contact offenders have less empathy for victims than Internet offenders and are also overly assertive, feel they are not in control of their lives, and display signs of impulsiveness.

Based on the data the authors evaluated, they believe that Internet offenders are unlikely to commit future contact sexual offenses. However, the authors of an article in a 2009 issue of the *Journal of Family Violence* found evidence that Internet offenders and contact offenders may be very similar. In this study, the authors collected data on convicted sexual offenders who were in a sex offender–specific residential treatment program. Seventy-four percent of the offenders had no documented cases of hands-on offending. They had been convicted of charges related to possession, receiving, or distributing child pornography. Twenty-four percent of the offenders in the treatment program had been convicted of hands-on sexual offenses.

By the end of the treatment program, 85 percent of the offenders had admitted to committing at least one hands-on offense. Many of these offenders simply had not been caught. They admitted their guilt during their treatment program. Only 15 percent of the offenders still maintained they never committed a hands-on act. Unfortunately, these offenders then were given a lie-detector test. Only two people passed, indicating the rest were still lying about having any hands-on involvement. Finally, the authors question whether or not there is much difference between child pornographers, child abusers, and pedophiles.

Restrictions

Convicted sex offenders living in some communities have restrictions placed on their Internet activities. For example, New York State has a law where convicted sex offenders must provide their information on their Internet accounts, including usernames for any networking Web sites. Of course, it is difficult to enforce such restrictions due to the inability to supervise a person's every movement.

CHILD PORNOGRAPHY

The Internet has made it very easy for people to share child pornography, which is any image or video form of pornography that involves children. Conservative estimates indicate that there are at least

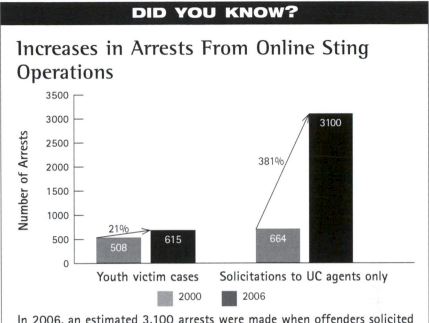

DID YOU KNOW?

Increases in Arrests From Online Sting Operations

In 2006, an estimated 3,100 arrests were made when offenders solicited undercover agents posing as children for sex. This was a 381 percent increase since 2000. Only 615 arrests were made when offenders solicited an actual child for sex, which was a 21 percent increase since 2000.

Source: *Trends in Arrests of Online Predators.* Crimes Against Children Research Center, 2009.

100,000 Web sites where people can find and share child pornography. Further, the use of peer-to-peer (P2P) technology allows people to share child pornography in a way that is unmonitored.

There are many documented cases where offenders have been arrested for sharing child pornography. The organization Stop Child Predators discusses several cases. In their 2009 online article, several notorious cases were documented. For example, in 2009, a man in Hawaii was arrested for having child pornography on his computer. Much of it was obtained using P2P file-sharing. Worse, he produced videos and images where young children were sexually assaulted.

Authors of a 2005 article in the journal *Swiss Medical Weekly* studied offenders convicted of having child pornography. The authors found that 42 percent of offenders had pictures depicting **pedophilia**. Another 18 percent had pictures of pedophilia, sadomasochism, and sodomy. The remaining 40 percent had different combinations of pictures related to pedophilia, sadomasochism, sodomy, and copro-philia.

A 2007 study in the journal *Sex Abuse* also looked at the collection and use of child pornography by Internet offenders. Approximately half of the offenders had paid for pictures of child pornography. The number of pictures found on an offender's computer ranged from two to 921,000. The average number of pictures was 16,698, a very large number only because some of the offenders had extensive collections. Another measure indicated that the average offender had 317 pictures at the time of arrest.

Q & A

Question: Does viewing pornography make sexual predators more dangerous?

Answer: The evidence indicates there is a relationship between the use of pornography and sexual aggression. Authors of a 2009 article in the *Journal of the American Psychiatric Nurses Association* found the use of pornography by juvenile sex offenders was a risk factor for sexual aggression. In an article found in a 2006 issue of the *Journal of Abnormal Psychology,* the authors found that offenders charged with possession of child pornography were more likely to meet the psychological criteria for pedophilia. However, the evidence linking pornography to sexual aggression is not concrete. The authors of an article in a 2009 issue of *Aggression and Violent Behavior* reviewed studies on the link between pornography and sexual aggression and argued that the evidence does not yet exist to say there is a certain relationship between the two.

Who are the victims?

Authors of an article in a 2007 issue of *Psychology, Crime & Law* also studied Internet sex offenders. The offenders in this study, all of whom were male, had been convicted of Internet sex offenses. Slightly more than 83 percent of the offenders indicated they had primarily viewed images of female children. Ages of the victims ranged from infant to older teenagers. The authors found that offenders had spent almost 12 hours per week viewing child pornography. Further, 50 percent of the offenders were found to have been viewing images that were considered the "most serious" of offensive pictures. At the time of arrest, offenders had between one and 51,000 images on their computers.

SEX OFFENDERS AND ONLINE BEHAVIOR

The author of a 2007 study in the *Journal of Child Sexual Abuse* studied how sex offenders identified and contacted minors over the Internet and found that 81 percent of the offenders used chat rooms to find children and teenagers. Almost 49 percent of offenders also reviewed online profiles, while 9.7 percent indicated they screened bulletin board postings. Offenders would look at screen names and the comments of users. If either made any reference to sex, that would catch the attention of offenders. If a screen name possibly indicated the user was young, that also would catch a predator's attention.

Fifty-two percent of offenders, after having made contact, would send pictures of child pornography to the kids they spoke with. Ninety-seven percent had explicitly sexual online conversations with the minors they wanted to meet. Finally, 29 percent represented themselves as children during their conversations.

How predators think

A 2008 study in the *Howard Journal* presented findings on how a pedophile thinks. The authors of this study extensively interviewed a convicted pedophile. Part of their interview focused on how the offender used the Internet. This person believed the Internet is designed for sexual thoughts. In this case the offender did not use the Internet to search out potential victims. The offender had access to victims without the need to find them online. However, the ability to find child pornography helped fuel fantasies of having sexual relations with children.

Avoiding detection

In an effort to avoid detection, offenders have adopted countersurveillance strategies. A 2009 article published in the *International Journal of Technology and Human Interactions* presented information on such strategies. The author interviewed offenders convicted of possessing child pornography. The author found that offenders used both technological and social strategies. The key technological strategy predators use is to secure connections and encryption techniques. The offenders felt that unsecured Web sites or unencrypted file-sharing could easily be intercepted.

Social strategies used by predators to avoid being caught include using aliases and not revealing personal information. Even when secure connections are used, there is a feeling that if one offender is caught he will share information about other offenders. Another strategy used was to vary patterns of behavior. One offender indicated that downloading different amounts of material and using a variety of Web sites helps obscure patterns. As encounters with Internet predators can be dangerous, it is important to understand what they search for and avoid releasing unnecessary personal information.

See also: Chat Rooms and Instant Messaging; Internet Safety; Online Predators, Characteristics of; Screen Names

FURTHER READING
Salter, Anna. *Predators: Pedophiles, Rapists, and Other Sex Offenders.* Jackson, Tenn.: Basic Books, 2004.
Sax, Robin. *Predators and Child Molesters: What Every Parent Needs to Know to Keep Kids Safe.* Amherst, N.Y.: Prometheus Books, 2009.
Wright, Richard. *Sex Offender Laws: Failed Policies, New Directions.* New York: Springer Publishing Company, 2009.

■ SOCIAL NETWORKING BEHAVIORS
See: Social Networking Web Sites

■ SOCIAL NETWORKING WEB SITES
Online locations designed for social interaction. Social networking Web sites, such as Friendster, Facebook, and MySpace, allow people to interact with each other through the Internet. Users create profiles and invite other users to join their personal network. Facebook is the most popular social networking site, followed by MySpace. Online social networks are seen as an extension of in-person social networks.

SOCIAL NETWORKING HISTORY
You may be surprised to learn that social networking sites were in existence long before MySpace or Facebook became popular. An online article found on digitaltrends.com discusses earlier versions, including BBS, America Online, and CompuServe. BBS stands for bul-

letin board system. A bulletin board system resembled what is known as a chat group today. People could post messages for other people. However, a BBS was a text-based system and often had a clunky interface. The digitaltrends article points out that people could upload and download programs. It was similar to what one currently finds on BitTorrent Web sites. Although bulletin board systems are considered archaic now, they were once very popular.

More advanced versions of a BBS were introduced during the 1980s. Two common examples are Delphi and CompuServe. Delphi was a paid service. People would dial a local access number that would connect them to the service. Similar to a BBS, people could post public comments and exchange files. People also could send private messages to each other, a rudimentary form of e-mail. As with bulletin board systems, Delphi was completely text-based.

The most popular service that resembled modern social networking was CompuServe. The company was founded in 1969 with the goal of providing computer time-sharing services to companies, as well as providing computer support for a life insurance company (Golden United Life Insurance, Inc.). During the 1980s, it became one of the largest networking services in the United States. Similar to bulletin board systems and Delphi, people could exchange information in public forums and send private messages. There were thousands of discussion forums, each dealing with a specific topic. CompuServe charged people an hourly fee to use its service before switching to a monthly subscription rate. By 1995, the company had more than 3 million subscribers.

American Online (AOL) became *the* online service during the 1990s. The company's history dates back into the 1980s; however, it was in the early 1990s that the company introduced a widespread service that incorporated social networking features. One benefit of AOL was its graphics interface. Gone were the days of text-only services. The company was able to take advantage of improved versions of both Windows and Macintosh operating systems. In many regards, AOL was the Internet before the Internet became common. Most people would use AOL for all of their online needs. Another benefit of AOL was they introduced real-time chat rooms. People could talk to each other without the delays associated with e-mail and online forums. America Online is still in service today.

From a historical perspective, it is easier to see how these services had social networking components. By today's standards, however, they would not be considered social networks.

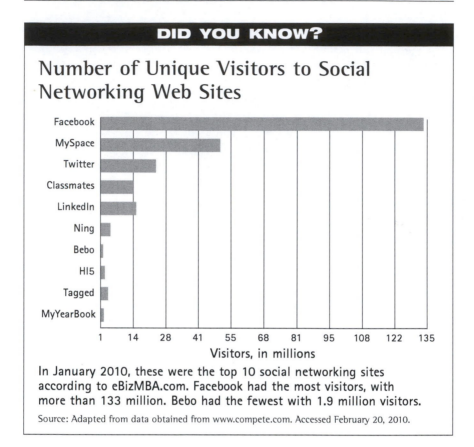

DID YOU KNOW?

Number of Unique Visitors to Social Networking Web Sites

In January 2010, these were the top 10 social networking sites according to eBizMBA.com. Facebook had the most visitors, with more than 133 million. Bebo had the fewest with 1.9 million visitors.

Source: Adapted from data obtained from www.compete.com. Accessed February 20, 2010.

FRIENDSTER

Friendster is one of the first "true" social networking Web sites. Friendster allows people to keep in touch with others, regardless of where they live. According to the company, there are more than 110 million users. As with other social networking Web sites discussed here, users can invite others to be part of their friendship network. A person can seek out others by searching for a variety of criteria: age, gender, location, college, high school, and more.

FACEBOOK

Facebook is considered the premiere social networking site. In 2004, a Harvard student named Mark Zuckerberg designed what was known at the time as thefacebook. The original goal of Facebook was to allow students to keep in touch and learn more about each other. At

first it was limited to just Harvard students. However, the Web site's popularity grew so fast that the service was expanded to other colleges. Within two years, the general public could also use Facebook.

Facebook's popularity continues to grow. According to comScore, a company that tracks online behavior for marketing purposes, in December 2008 there were 54.5 million unique visitors to the Web site. The company says that in December 2009 there were almost 112 million unique visitors. The number of visitors grew by 105 percent.

A 2010 report by Hitwise indicates that for the week ending January 23, Facebook accounted for 48.09 percent of all visits to a social networking site. The Nielsen Company, in a 2010 report, found that for the previous month (December 2009), the average number of visits to Facebook per user was 51. On average a person spent slightly more than six hours during the month on Facebook. That comes out to a little more than two hours per day.

A short article that appeared on the Web site eBizMBA ranked the 20 most popular social networking Web sites. According to information they obtained, Facebook was the number one ranked social networking site. According to this report, an estimated 122 million people used Facebook in December 2009.

Facebook has taken social networking to a new level. In addition to connecting with other people, a user can play numerous online games. This includes competing against others to see who can obtain the highest score. People can upload photos for others to look at. A user can search for people around the country and the world.

Users control how much information other people see. Settings allow users to let everyone on Facebook see all information to only letting certain friends see specific information. The user controls access to information at all times. An excellent benefit is that Facebook can help prevent unknown people from learning about a user, depending on the privacy settings.

For some people this security feature is meaningless. A person who allows the public to view all information is exposing himself or herself to potential problems, such as strangers possibly learning more than they should.

Also, some Facebook users have thousands of friends. They accept anyone who requests to add them as a friend. This can become the equivalent of allowing all personal information to be public. A person cannot be completely sure that others are honest.

MYSPACE

Another dominant force in social networking is MySpace. MySpace has been around since January 2004. MySpace, in a sense, was an evolution of Friendster. Several users of Friendster saw the potential to do more with social networking. According to comScore, as of January 2010 there were approximately 70 million MySpace users in the United States.

MySpace has many of the same features found on Facebook. Users can search out other people, play games, upload pictures, share information about themselves, listen to music, and much more. In many ways MySpace is more flexible than Facebook, because users can customize how their profiles look, including changing background images and incorporating music. That makes a profile look more personal and can help reveal someone's personality. Unfortunately, many profiles become almost impossible to read because of picture and color combinations.

For a while, MySpace was the top social networking site. It gained so much popularity among teens that adults started to worry about the safety of the Web site. There have been high profile cases where Internet predators were caught trying to meet children through MySpace. Media coverage of such arrests have fueled parents' concerns about MySpace. However, MySpace is no more dangerous than other social networking Web sites.

TWITTER

Twitter is a unique form of social networking. Unlike Facebook or MySpace, there are not many features to Twitter. Instead, Twitter allows people to post short remarks, referred to as tweets. A tweet can be no longer than 140 characters. Users can type in anything they want and that information can instantly be shared with others.

In order to receive tweets from other people, a person has to become a follower. Unlike Facebook a person does not need permission to be a follower. As a user you can follow as many people as you want. Of course, a user can prevent another person from reading his or her tweets.

Twitter was founded in 2006 and quickly became an online hit. According to a 2009 report by Compete.com, Twitter went from being the 22nd most visited social networking site at the beginning of 2008 to the third most visited by January 2009. It experienced a **1,227 percent growth in 12 months.**

Q & A

Question: Is Twitter considered social networking or blogging?

Answer: There is no clear answer to that question. It is typically considered a social networking Web site. However, it can also be viewed as micro-blogging. People post short comments about what they are doing, how they feel, what is on their mind, and so forth. For children and teenagers, it does not seem to matter what Twitter is, because data indicate that most children and teens do not use it. A 2010 study by the Pew Research Center found that only 8 percent of teens use Twitter.

OTHER SOCIAL NETWORKING WEB SITES

The Web sites discussed above are among the most popular social networking sites in the country. However, there are countless other social networking sites in existence. They may be general sites where people can post information about anything. They may be specific sites, such as LinkedIn, which focuses on cultivating business relationships.

According to a list provided by eBizMBA.com, in December 2010 the following Web sites were the 15 most popular social networking sites:

1. Facebook
2. MySpace
3. Twitter
4. LinkedIn
5. Ning
6. Tagged
7. Classmates
8. HI5
9. Myyearbook
10. Meetup
11. Bebo
12. Mylife
13. Friendster
14. myHeritage
15. Multiply

SOME CONCLUSIONS

Social networking Web sites provide people with opportunities to have meaningful interactions with others. The Web sites themselves are not risky. Risk is a factor only when users decide how much information they share and with whom.

See also: Blogging; Bullies and Cyber-bullying; Chat Rooms and Instant Messaging; Internet Safety; Screen Names; Surfing and Online Communication

FURTHER READING

Awl, Dave. *Facebook Me! A Guide to Having Fun With Your Friends and Promoting Your Projects on Facebook.* Berkeley, Calif.: Peachpit Press, 2009.

Christakis, Nicholas A., and James H. Fowler. *Connected: The Surprising Power of Our Social Networks and How They Shape Our Lives.* New York: Little, Brown and Company, 2009.

Hannon, Matt. *The Smart Parent's Guide to Facebook: Easy Tips to Protect and Connect With Your Teen.* Charleston, S.C.: CreateSpace, 2009.

■ SURFING AND ONLINE COMMUNICATION

Using the Internet to find information and communicating with others in a proper manner. Online users should follow the rules of **netiquette,** or Internet etiquette. Users should act responsibly online. In addition to being polite to others during online communication, users should limit the amount of personal information they share. This can help reduce the likelihood of being victimized.

WHAT IS SURFING?

Surfing is a term that was coined in 1992 by Jean Armour Polly. On Polly's Web site, Netmom.com, she discusses how she came up with the term. At the time, she was writing an article on using the Internet and was looking for a term that would describe the fun she had online. She also wanted a word that would "evoke a sense of randomness, chaos, and even danger." According to Polly, at the time she was using a mouse pad that had a surfer on a wave with the words *Information Surfer* on it. She drew from that and came up with surfing. The term has been around ever since.

NETIQUETTE

As the Internet rapidly grew in popularity, various rules started to develop. These guidelines focused on the proper way to interact with others through the Internet. The term netiquette refers to Internet etiquette. One of the first set of rules was published by Virginia Shea in *The Core Rules of Netiquette* in 1994. These core rules have not changed and still make up the basis for interacting with others in an appropriate manner.

Shea lists 10 rules:

1. Remember the human.
2. Adhere to the same standards of behavior online that you follow in real life.
3. Know where you are in cyberspace.
4. Respect other people's time and bandwidth.
5. Make yourself look good online.
6. Share expert knowledge.
7. Help keep flame wars under control.
8. Respect other people's privacy.
9. Don't abuse your power.
10. Be forgiving of other people's mistakes.

These rules apply to both the real world and the Internet. There are only a couple of rules that need to be expanded on. Rule 3, "know where you are in cyberspace," refers to the fact that different rules may apply to different aspects of online behavior. It also can refer to the fact that different rules may apply to different chat rooms. The type of discussions that are acceptable in one room may differ in another room.

Rule 9, "don't abuse your power," means not to take advantage of situations. In particular, Shea was referring to online games where some users may be more powerful than others. She also mentioned that some users may have more computer administrative privileges than others, and those privileges should not be abused.

There are also several rules when it comes to e-mail etiquette. Sending spam or junk e-mail is in poor taste and usually will make the recipients angry. Junk filters for e-mail help to greatly reduce the amount of spam that arrives in a person's inbox. However, it is still offensive and illegal.

It is also recommended that users not send e-mails with attachments unless the recipient is expecting it. Given the problems with computer viruses, many users will not even read an e-mail that arrives with an attachment. It is recommended that the recipient be notified first about the attachment and then send it once permission has been granted.

Offensive, abusive, and profane e-mails are inappropriate. They can constitute harassment, which can prompt a visit from the authorities if the e-mail is abusive or threatening. Also, writing in all capital letters is frowned upon. Not only does it make reading a message more difficult, it is viewed as yelling at the reader. Using large or small fonts is also inappropriate. A 10 to 14 point font is acceptable, depending on the style of the font used.

Another aspect of online communication is the use of "netlingo," abbreviations of words. Using abbreviations cuts down on the time needed to send messages, and they are very common in both chat rooms and when sending text messages. However, it is not recommended that these be used unless the reader knows what the abbreviations mean. When sending e-mails netlingo should not be used unless the e-mail is being sent to a friend or family member. Using netlingo when sending formal e-mails, such as to a teacher, is inappropriate. It is the equivalent of using slang when talking to someone. For informal use, the Web site Netlingo.com has a detailed list of abbreviations used for chat and text messages.

BEING RESPONSIBLE

Being responsible goes beyond being respectful to others online. It also means minimizing the chances of being victimized in some manner. Because the Internet is used by offenders to help steal identities, e-mail, blogs, chat rooms, and instant messaging software creates opportunities for people to harass each other. This means that people need to think about what information they will share with others. Personal information can be used against someone or may help an offender identify where a person lives, works, or goes to school. Although social networking Web sites and blogs are designed so people can learn about others, discretion should be used when it comes to personal information. Just like in the physical world, it is better to be safe than sorry.

See also: Bullies and Cyber-bullying; Internet Safety; Peers and Peer Pressure; Prejudice and Online Behavior; Screen Names; Social Networking Web sites

FURTHER READING

Cimino, Michelle. *NETiquette (On-line Etiquette): Tips for Adults & Teens: Facebook, MySpace, Twitter! Terminology . . . and More.* Frederick, Md.: PublishAmerica, 2009.

Donelan, Helen, Karen Kear, and Magnus Ramage. *Online Communication and Collaboration: A Reader.* Florence, Ky.: Routledge, 2010.

▓ TEXTING
See: Bullies and Cyber-bullying; Chat Rooms and Instant Messaging

▓ TWITTER
See: Prevalence and Statistics; Social Networking Web Sites

HOTLINES AND HELP SITES

Anti-Phishing Working Group (APWG)
URL: http://www.antiphishing.org
Program: The Anti-Phishing Working Group is an industry association focused on eliminating the identity theft and fraud that result from the growing problem of phishing and e-mail spoofing. The organization provides a forum to discuss phishing issues, define the scope of the phishing problem in terms of hard and soft costs, and share information and best practices for eliminating the problem. Where appropriate, the APWG shares this information with law enforcement.

Federal Trade Commission (FTC)
URL: http://www.ftc.gov
Phone: (877) ID-THEFT
Program: The Federal Trade Commission investigates complaints related to identity theft. It also provides resources for questions about Internet privacy issues.

National Center for Missing and Exploited Children.
URL: http://www.missingkids.com
Phone: (800) 843-5678
Program: The NCMEC provides resources related to the issues of missing and exploited children.

National Center for Victims of Crime
URL: http://www.ncvc.org
Phone: (800) FYI-CALL
Program: The NCVC provides help and resources to people who have
   been victimized by all types of crime.

National Fraud Information Hotline
URL: http://www.fraud.org
Phone: (800) 876-7060
Programs: Allows fraud victims to file a complaint; the hotline also
   has resources to learn more about different types of fraud.

GLOSSARY

avatar a two- or three-dimensional image that is used on the Internet to represent the user

censoring banning or deleting information to prevent others from seeing it

child pornography sexually explicit images involving children

computer viruses *see* viruses

cookies computer code that is used to track a person's movements on the Internet

cyber-crime crimes committed using computers, computer networks, and the Internet

cybersex sexual behavior that occurs over the Internet

download information transferred from a computer or server to a user's computer

drive-by pharming occurs when malicious code is placed on a user's computer, altering the user's Internet settings

dysphoria general feeling of depression or distress that is characterized by anxiety, uneasiness, restlessness, or agitation

e-mail spoofing fraudulent activity that involves changing the appearance of an e-mail so it seems to come from a legitimate person or institution

firewall program or device that prevents a person's computer from being accessed by others over the Internet

flaming insulting or harassing comments made between users in chat rooms, social forums, e-mails, or instant messages

grooming behavior that establishes a connection with a child in order to facilitate sexual abuse

hardware physical components of a computer

identity theft fraudulently obtaining personal information to access financial accounts

invisible content hidden information inserted into a phishing e-mail and used to bypass spam filters

libel using the written word, false accusations, or misrepresentations of a person

malicious code *see* **malware**

malware computer code designed to gain access to a computer without the user's permission

mimicry behavior that is imitative

netiquette shortened version of *internet etiquette;* refers to behaving in a civil manner when interacting with others through the Internet

pedophilia perverse sexual attraction to children

peer pressure the influence that one's peers have over a person's behavior

privacy negotiations privacy tradeoffs a person makes when using a free social networking Web site

privacy priming (privacy salience) negative effects privacy policies can have on information sharing

private browsing option found in many Web browsers that prevents the software from collecting or retaining information

pseudonym fictitious or false name used by a person, often to protect that person's real identity

public domain intellectual property that is not protected by copyright laws and can be used by anyone

reference group group of people who are equal in one's age and social standing; peers

search engine Web site that retrieves information based on search criteria

slippery slope argument belief that a course of action will lead to further actions with unintended consequences

social engineering manipulating people into providing information that is typically confidential

social networking online interaction between people that leads to the creation of Internet communities

software programs that tell a computer what to do

spam unsolicited and unwanted e-mails that are sent in bulk to users

spyware form of malware that collects information and actions without a user's consent

text messaging interacting with others via text on a cell phone

uploading   occurs when a user transfers a program to another computer or network

URL hiding   situation in which a hyperlink is provided in an e-mail that looks legitimate but directs the user to a fraudulent Web site

viruses   malware that can typically reproduce or replicate itself and cause harm to computers and networks

Web browser   software that allows people to use the Internet

INDEX

Boldface page numbers indicate extensive treatment of a topic.